THE
DIET
CODE

THE
DIET
CODE

REVOLUTIONARY WEIGHT LOSS SECRETS FROM DA VINCI AND THE GOLDEN RATIO

STEPHEN LANZALOTTA

Foreword by Walter B. Goldfarb, MD

WARNER WELLNESS

NEW YORK   BOSTON

Epilogue: Robert Gibbons, author of *Body of Time* (Pittsburgh: Mise Publications, 2004)

Warner Wellness

Warner Books
Time Warner Book Group
1271 Avenue of the Americas, New York, NY 10020
Visit our Web site at www.twbookmark.com.

Warner Wellness and the Warner Wellness logo are trademarks of Time Warner Book Group Inc.

Printed in the United States of America

First Edition: April 2006
10 9 8 7 6 5 4 3 2 1

ISBN-10: 0-446-57887-8
ISBN-13: 978-0-446-57887-5

Library of Congress Control Number: 2005937631

Book design by Giorgetta Bell McRee

Dedication

ДЛЯЖЕНИ

Chekhov observed, "If you love, you will die;
but if you don't love, you will die anyway."

Beyond what's necessary, you give me
the strength to do what's right

ACKNOWLEDGMENTS

Thank you David Sharp and Ryan Lenz, AP journalists, and Dave Weller at Random House for noticing this material and "getting the ball rolling."

Thanks to my parents, Ellen and Vin Lanzalotta, and to my family—immediate and ancestral—for generating "the ball."

To my mentors—Sheila Serrie and Wally Harris; Chief E. Tantaquidgeon; Wm. Coperthwaite; H. O'More; and Sensei C. Merriman—for "passing the ball" through four decades: fusing my education in natural sciences; the arts of native America, ancient Russia and the Mongolian steppe; Celtic and Grail lore; and Oriental martial arts.

To John, Flo, Ian, and Geoff—my "brothers in arms" for refusing to let me fail.

To my "goddesses"—M., Mandy, *and* Mandy, Shy, Sherry, Olivia, Nikki, and Veronika for a rebound net woven of eight directions.

To Aaiyn the maternal watcher.

To Mary at *Simply* for fax.

To the workers at Federal St. Post Office, Portland ME; and the good folks at *Java Net Café* for fielding months of manuscript packets and computer printouts.

To the extended family of *Micucci Italian Grocery* for their concern, cheerleading, and care with the deli orders.

To Rick and Lisa for their loyalty and patience with my insanity.

To Robert and Kathleen for research, wine in stormy weather, and for restating that "work is a form of worship."

To Jay and Liz, combining sushi and Yiddish humor into an elixir for tracking straight.

Thanks to Nicole. Coffee clutches, companionship, and her tireless computer slogging allowed me to meet deadlines. That you'll be reading these pages is thanks to Nicole.

To my kids who ate everything and actually approved it. And who shouldered a lot of responsibility when I was less of a dad and more of a recluse writer. I love you Seth, Shaia and Jari.

To my co-writer, Colleen Kapklein, agents Marly Rusoff and Michael Radulescu, and Janis Vallely, and editor Diana Baroni, for never losing faith even though I did.

To my bakery patrons whose enthusiasm remains after the most infuriatingly erratic hours of any dealer in dough since Gennaro Lombardi's a century ago.

To y'all; cuz thanks to those folks above yer gettin' somethin' good!

CONTENTS

FOREWORD

Steve Lanzalotta is a man of many talents, with a multifaceted approach to life that would make da Vinci himself proud. He's an artist working in many media, first and foremost dough.

I've been enjoying the fruits of his labor for a long time at his superb bakery café, Sophia's, and I've brought many of my medical colleagues and friends with me. So I was excited to discover he'd turned his talents to putting pen to paper to create a book—the book you now hold in your hands. For years I'd been happily eating and sharing pizza made from scratch, Italian salami on peasant bread, almond crusted flaky *girelle* pastries and, my favorite in the midst of a Maine winter, tomato and basil soup. Imagine my pleasure at hearing Steve make the case that this food was not only delicious and satisfying, but also naturally healthful and precisely proportioned for outstanding nutrition. The deal was sweetened by the prospect of being able to re-create the same food at home. The capper: hearing that many have used a plan based around these foods to lose weight and improve their health. Sold!

And so I offer my ringing endorsement of *The Diet Code* and its food. But if Steve becomes too successful, what are we long-standing aficionados going to do for lunch?

Steve's an Old World guy; one look at him and you'd think you were in Naples—the stubble, the apron, the flour all over his hands.

Step inside Sophia's, as I do a couple times a week, and you'll feel the warmth from the ovens, hear jazz over the sound system and see the owner's paintings on the walls. Don't even get me started on the heavenly smell—for that you don't even need to come inside, as it wafts down the street defying anyone to pass by fresh baked bread.

All that creates marvelous ambiance, but none of it would mean anything if the taste and authenticity of the food didn't deliver on the promise. And deliver it does. This is whole, natural Mediterranean-style cuisine at its simplest and best. I've not found better anywhere in Italy, from Liguria to Tuscany to Sicily, where I've seen for myself how Italians enjoy their food—wine, bread, pasta and pastries included—without any sign of the ever-expanding waistlines of Americans. I recently brought a box of Sophia's treats to an Italian friend, who lifted the lid, took one whiff of the pastry and said, "That's my grandmother's!" I can think of no better testament to the quality and authenticity of the magic of Steve's food. What's not to love about a "diet" plan based around that?

I'm a firm believer that the lifestyle one leads in the 22 hours a day that one is *not* eating is as important as exactly what you ingest in the other two. With food like this, though, you know you're doing right by your body. Making good choices in both food and lifestyle, as this book recommends, you'll be doing as da Vinci did—and the Italians still do. I'm grateful to be able to experience a little piece of Italy and the Renaissance every time I'm in Steve's place. And glad readers everywhere will be able to bring the same experience into their homes with *The Diet Code*.

—Walter B. Goldfarb, MD
Portland, Maine
October 2005

Part I

UNDERSTANDING THE CODE

CHAPTER ONE

Leonardo da Vinci, the Golden Ratio—and What's for Dinner

The wisest and noblest teacher is nature itself.
—LEONARDO DA VINCI

Man achieves the height of Wisdom when all that he does is as self-evident as what Nature does.
—I CHING

Milan, Winter 1492

The pencil drops from Leonardo's left hand as he picks up a chunk of bigio, or whole grain bread, to soak up broth from a steaming bowl of minestra, a Milanese broth featuring the region's distinctive savoy cabbage and a mix of root vegetables and their greens. He distractedly stabs at a bit of turnip with the fork in his right hand. Within reach are some thin slabs of creamy Taleggio cheese and a flask of wine from the vineyards of his patron, Ludovico Sforza, duke of Bari.

Momentarily focusing on his soup, Leonardo reminisces about his native Tuscany and the Florentine minestrone, spicy and meaty from a soffrito mix of minced and sautéed chicken giblets, pork and peppercorns. The duke had been suitably surprised by the dish when Leonardo prepared it for him. The Lombard ruler is quite fond of meat from the pig and well knows of Leonardo's reputation as a brilliant cook, but it was the last meal he expected from a vegetarian's kitchen.

Leonardo isn't painting much these days, because the duke is presently more interested in civic planning and engineering—moats, walls, *war machines and the like. But the duke has been suggesting a fresco for the Dominican monastery of Santa Maria delle Grazie, and Leonardo is already plotting the depiction of another meal of bread and wine. Unbeknownst to his patron, the artist has in mind to use the fresco to convey a message so grand, so unexpected and so shocking that its deepest meanings will have to be encoded if the fresco is to be painted at all.*

That will come later, though. Now, Leonardo occupies his peripatetic mind with plotting the geometry of what will become one of his greatest works. Lifting the bowl to sip the last of his soup, he contemplates proportioning the enormous work by what he calls secto d'aurea—*golden section or, as it is later renamed, the golden ratio. He visualizes the way lines will relate to each other, forming key angles. If the numbers governing the structure of a painting are right, he knows, the aesthetic will resonate deep within viewers.*

Leonardo lifts the bowl to his lips, sips the last of his soup and mops up the final drops with a crust torn from the loaf, enjoying a secret latent in his lunch: the key to long life and good health is literally in his hands.

In this imagined scene, one of the world's great geniuses finishes a meal as ideally proportioned as any of his master works. What Leonardo da Vinci brought *a tavolo* (to the table) was as balanced as anything he consciously designed during his long career—a career in which he devoted much energy to exploring and exploiting an ancient mathematical formula that's come to be known as the Golden Ratio. Leonardo's application of the Golden Ratio was arguably quite calculated when it came to his art, but it was likely intuitive when it came to his meal planning. Leonardo simply chose from the variety of fresh whole foods available to him, nourishing his body and mind with ease in a way we seem to have entirely abandoned today. The effect of proper proportions is just as powerful on the plate and in the body, however, as it is on a canvas. Leonardo dined on the particular ancient triumvirate of bread, wine and cheese, which makes up the trinity of essential macronutrients—carbohydrate, protein and fat.

Leonardo, for one, reaped the benefits. He was slender throughout his long life and famously strong. (He was said to be capable of bending horseshoes with a single hand or stopping a horse running past him at full gallop with his bare hands.) That's not to mention cultivating perhaps the most amazing brain ever—one of the keenest, most synthetic and far-reaching intellects of all time!

While I can't guarantee that eating the same way will turn you into a great painter, inventor, architect, engineer, botanist, anatomist, astronomer or sculptor, I *can* promise that consciously re-creating the quality, combinations and proportion of foods Leonardo relied on will help you become lean and strong. Put these new proportions inside your body, and you'll soon see new proportions outside. All you have to do is crack The Diet Code—master the simple formula that unlocks the secret to easy weight loss: maximizing nutrition and metabolism.

—m—

As a self-taught baker raised on my grandmother's rustic Italian cooking, I've thrived on meals much like those on which Leonardo must have supped. I make breads hardly different from those he would have known, using the exact same technology as bakers in Leonardo's time did. More directly, I've admired Leonardo's polymath mind and strived for decades to take what insights I could from him and apply them across multiple aspects of my life. Again and again, I've circled back to that one formula, famously encoded in the angles of his spread-eagle *Vitruvian Man,* among many of his other works, not to mention a litany of designs dating back to the earliest human civilizations: the Golden Ratio.

The Golden Ratio guided Leonardo in designing the famous fresco (*The Last Supper*) that I imagine him contemplating in the opening of this chapter and has been given credit for the enthralling effect of his

Mona Lisa. He used it in his more practical undertakings, too, proportioning garden schematics, city planning layouts, everyday engineering plans and the like. In doing so, he was rediscovering wisdom from ancient Rome, Greece, Egypt and Mesopotamia, which had at that point been all but lost; among Leonardo's many extraordinary achievements count rescuing and revitalizing this vital knowledge.

The latest cutting-edge science and technology has proven just how deep this mathematical wisdom goes, documenting the Golden Ratio in everything from the pattern of galaxies and the shape of ocean waves to the spiral of seashells and the arrangement of petals in a rose. The same natural laws of design also dictate the form of human genetic material (the DNA double helix), the development of the human fetus and many details in the architecture of the human body. The Golden Ratio has been successfully applied by humans in so many arenas simply because they affirm the greater wisdom of nature when they do so.

This ancient formula has guided *me* in designing my own woodworking tools as well as whatever I create with those tools. The Golden Ratio gets credit for the impact of my abstract paintings, even fixating people who don't "like" modern art. As I later turned to bread making, what I'd learned about ideal proportions and numerical, geometric and mathematical relationships helped me perfect the breads I turn out daily at my bakery café.

And now, after decades of experimenting with applications like these, gradually extending the use of the Golden Ratio into new aspects of my life, it's finally impressed me most in the most mundane area: what I eat. I learned to use the same "magic" that perfected my tools and keeps my bread in such demand to balance my diet and fuel my body better than I'd ever done before. In tinkering with the Golden Ratio, I've discovered it describes the diet that is most closely aligned with the needs of the human body, providing foods and nutrients in the exact proportions that dictate the inherent design of the body. Once I'd figured out how to use the numbers this way, it seemed it should have been obvious: The food that's best for the body is the food that follows the same blueprint as does the human body. *Of course* the same formula that dictates how you are put together should also dictate how you feed yourself. And when it does, you are working in harmony with your body's systems, and the natural result is optimal health and ideal weight.

Beyond that, a diet laid out in the Golden Ratio meets—in fact, exceeds—all accepted nutritional standards. It also looks gorgeous on the plate, tastes amazing and satisfies completely. And it stabilized my weight right where it was while I was a high school football player, even as I hit my mid-40s! All that, plus I can fix dinner in less than half an hour. *And* my children will devour it.

—⚅—

Drawing on this same formula, The Diet Code is a complete, balanced, satisfying and sane way to eat. And the only thing it has you do without entirely is the denial and extremes of fad diets. It is the feeling of deprivation that makes fad diets—even those on which many find short-term success—unsustainable. The Diet Code is flexible enough to encompass what *you* like to eat. This plan can be followed by vegans, vegetarians or those who, like me, enjoy a good steak. If you like wine or beer with your dinner, that fits in, too. You can indulge your sweet tooth (I'll show you how) without fear of undermining your results. Yes, you can fly in the face of recent decades of dietary advice. Eat bread! Eat butter! With its unique, proportional harmony between food groups and practical advice distilled into plans for truly balanced meals that are as simple and quick to make as they are delicious, The Diet Code is perfect for a post-Atkins America.

But it's not meant to be a quick fix. Rather, The Diet Code is a lifetime plan that honors both the art and the science of eating well. It provides exacting information for maximizing metabolic power and nutritional impact while you luxuriate in the pure, sensual pleasure of eating truly good food—foods that are easily acquired and prepared to suit people living today's hectic lifestyles. Drawing on traditional Italian foods—and, as important, traditional Italian ways of cooking and eating—The Diet Code guides you toward freedom from food fads and fears with an Old World perspective that requires you to eat *for pleasure*.

The Diet Code allows you to lose weight at nutritionists' recommended rate for healthy, stable and permanent weight loss: 1–2 pounds a week; 4–8 pounds a month. You'll be eating so well that the weight loss will seem almost effortless. Over time, eating this way will restructure your metabolism and alkalize your system, creating vibrant good health as well as maintaining your natural, healthy weight.

I've experienced the changes that eating this way has brought about in my own body and have witnessed it working for others as they discovered it at my shop, Sophia's. When I made the transition to eating essentially this way (years before I fine-tuned it exactly to the Golden Ratio), the extra pounds I'd been carrying around fell away. Once I refined my personal practices precisely to match the Golden Ratio, I grew leaner still and more muscular. The numbers on the scale didn't really change, since muscle weighs more than fat, but I looked somehow less fleshy, and my clothes fit differently. Equally important, meals proportioned according to the Golden Ratio gave me the energy I needed—the baker's life is a physically demanding one.

As soon as I realized the power of combining foods this way in my own life, I designed a menu along the same lines to serve in my bakery café. My customers responded as enthusiastically as they always had to my bread and began asking how they could eat like this at home, too. And many reported losing weight.

One woman, for example, told me she had started on the South Beach Diet before switching over to The Diet Code approach. She then ate bread every day and still reached her original target weight on time, dropping 25 pounds in four months. She's now the perfect fit for one of the (size small) T-shirts I sell in my shop, the ones that brag "Body by Bread"!

Another woman in her 40s ate The Diet Code way during and after her recent pregnancy. Just recently she was in the store for a pizza with her family (including her three-month-old)—and back at her usual size 4, with no trace left of the 50 pounds she'd put on while pregnant.

A woman in her 60s came into the shop excited about her early success with the plan. "You might not be able to tell, since I'm still stout," she said to me, "but I've lost 7 pounds already!"

Even my own daughter, tall and slim but, in the unfortunate way of teenage girls everywhere, conscious of her weight, lost 7 pounds in three weeks when she started eating The Diet Code way. Since she wasn't overweight to begin with, her weight then stabilized. On both counts (the loss and the stabilization), *proportion* was the key. My daughter had been eating a typical American diet at her mom's— coffee cake for breakfast, mac and cheese for dinner—heavy on the starch, without the fresh vegetables and the balanced fat and protein to complement the carbs.

Even people who don't need or want to lose weight can reap the benefits of following The Diet Code. My son, who has that beanpole build many teenage boys specialize in, noticed a difference when he moved back in with me. Over dinner one night, he said, "Dad, have you noticed I haven't been sick in about a year and a half? I haven't even had a cold. That's never happened before!" One of my employees recently told me I saved his life—he no longer craved junk food once he started eating from my shop. Getting better nutrition as well as better taste, he said his body was just not happy when he ate anywhere else.

Now this book reveals a plan anyone can use to reap the same benefits my family, my customers and I have. As many times and as many ways as the Golden Ratio has been used through the ages, never before has it been applied to taking in foods and nutrients in proportion with the inherent design of the human body—and the universe. When your food is correctly selected, combined, portioned and proportioned to be directly in sync with your natural metabolic needs, the inevitable result is optimal health and ideal weight.

The Diet Code unlocks all that for you. This is age-old math, but revealed here for the first time is how it works with food, nutrition and weight loss. The Golden Ratio has kept artists and scholars busy exploring its complexities for millennia, yet in the end The Diet Code is as simple as one, two, three, as you'll discover in chapter 2. The basic weight loss formula is accessible to anyone and everyone. The Diet Code program consists of three stages, which I'll walk you through in chapter 7: a gentle initiation for beginners, including the specific formula for creating Diet Code meals; more details in a somewhat more intense period in the middle of the learning curve; and a final phase in which you relax into a lifetime of eating this way, having internalized the principles.

—⁓—

As I developed meals according to the Golden Ratio, I saw that not only was I using the numbers Leonardo did, I was using his foods, too. Not in the strictest sense, of course—tomatoes are a staple of mine, for example, but they weren't even introduced in Italy from the New World until near the end of Leonardo's lifetime, and I do eat meat, while he was a vegetarian for most of his adult life. Leonardo lived during a prosperous time in Italian history, in a financial and cultural capital of the world. Food was generally plentiful—certainly for tradesmen and the upper classes—and varied, thanks to a moderate climate, extensive agriculture and bustling worldwide trade. Food was also fresh, whole, organic, local, free-range, antibiotic-free, pesticide-free, unprocessed and nutrient-dense. General dietary patterns at the time reflect what I've now worked out as Golden Ratio proportions: carbohydrate based and balanced by moderate protein intake and the inclusion of healthy fats—Leonardo's lunch of bread, cheese and vegetable soup. For these reasons, I initially thought of the system I was working out as "the da Vinci diet," referencing not only the man and his math, but also the time (fifteenth century) and place in which he lived. His home village (Vinci) in the Tuscan hills was once ancient Etruria, a cultural and culinary center of Italy even before Roman civilization developed.

That seemingly simple meal fueled not just Leonardo's genius but also the genius of his whole era. He lived during the Renaissance, which saw unprecedented changes to Italy, Europe and the world. It was an awakening unlike any before or since; literally (in French, via

Latin) a rebirth. The fifteenth century was a maelstrom of rebirth of human aspirations, values and visions, a time of unrepentant inquiry in science, perspective, sociology and theology. It saw perhaps the biggest paradigm shift of all time, and everything was in play. It was a rebirth following a millennium of church domination during which scientific learning was suppressed and a dark age marked by traveling laborers, serfdom and ignorance was spread. It was also a rebirth after the Black Death wiped out one-third of the population of Europe.

RENAISSANCE MAN

Father of the submarine, bicycle, automobile, flying machine and computer, along with his fine art legacy, Leonardo da Vinci was the ultimate Renaissance man. The author Maria Costantino wrote that he was "possibly the most versatile genius in the history of mankind, consistently demonstrating ideas far ahead of his time. . . . Today both his scientific vision and his skill as an artist seem breathtaking."

Leonardo as a Renaissance man has particular personal meaning for me not in what he invented (wondrous though those are), but rather in what he ceaselessly strove to apply anew—having inherited knowledge from a long chain of people who'd gone before him. In the age of intrigue, suspicion and unrest in which he lived, everyone was on the move, often for their very lives. Counts and dukes wrangled for alliances; artists migrated from region to region seeking paying patrons. Little wonder Leonardo encoded and secreted his occult knowledge in enigmatic works that baffle us today.

Having struggled myself for decades against indoctrination and cultural biases to keep methods and teachings of the ancients alive amidst a fast-paced consumer-oriented present, I have come to respect Leonardo's persistence as much as or more than his creative genius.

With the invention of the printing press, mass media were born, beginning with the printing of the Bible. Trade routes to the East brought Chinese gunpowder and Islamic mathematics to Europe; firepower and more sophisticated calculations led to regular trans-Atlantic navigation and the subsequent plundering of the Americas. Society's entire worldview changed, quite literally, making possible the acceptance of Copernican theory (that the earth revolves around the sun, not vice versa) and the proposition that the globe is spherical. Scientists and scholars working from ancient Greek and Egyptian texts upset the canon of the clergy. Renaissance culture brought about breakthroughs in thought and advances in art, architecture, anatomy, cosmology, global navigation, engineering, humanism and social reform.

Taken together, this was one of the most significant clusters of events in human history, and it simultaneously expanded and fractured provincial Europe. Yet through this revolution, cuisine and culinary arts stayed much the same. What happened in the fields and at the tables of ordinary people may have been the only area of life not subjected to a major upheaval. Those ordinary people were working from truths with roots too strong to allow dislocation. The people of the Renaissance performed intense physical and mental exertions on a balanced base of carb-rich foods, including grains, beans, vegetables and fruits, combined judiciously with healthy fats and proteins. Leonardo and his fellow Tuscan *mangiafagioli* (bean eaters) would have been eating bread, pasta, wine and all kinds of fruits and vegetables, including leafy greens, onions, nuts and figs—from the whole, unadulterated and organic *dieta* (fare) available to him in the fifteenth century. Leonardo's diet was as much in rhythm with the design and function of the human body and the natural world around him as were his creative efforts.

—⁂—

You might say I'm a bit of a Renaissance man myself: abstract painter, master woodworker, amateur classical and jazz pianist and violinist, student of the martial arts—as well as baker and chef. And a single father with three teenagers. So I'm serious about the personal expression made possible through preparing wonderful food, and equally serious about making that a real-life proposition. Some nights, you just need to get a meal on the table. But even in the midst of a busy life, that meal can be a thing of beauty: gracefully proportioned aesthetically and nutritionally, and perfectly in sync with the needs of the healthy human body.

To that end, part I of this book examines the math behind the Golden Ratio and how I came to realize that a magical-seeming series of numbers held the secret to healthy eating and weight loss. It considers how out of balance our diets have become, as we've lost touch with the foods that have nurtured us and sustained us for almost the entirety of human history, and shows how crucial it is for us to reclaim what we've left behind.

Part II of the book presents the practical part of the program, giving you a closer look at the science behind and simple methods for living by The Diet Code. It includes a look at the problems with cutting any food group out of your diet—a mystifyingly popular approach guaranteed to result in a drastically imbalanced diet destined to cause weight gain and malnutrition simultaneously—and why the only food you need to avoid for weight loss success is *fake* food. One chapter describes the short list of Fundamental Foods at the heart of The Diet Code program and introduces how to apply the Golden Ratio to be sure you get them in the proportions necessary for weight loss. Another gives you the five basic steps you need to take to implement The Diet Code: choosing foods by asking yourself, *What would Leonardo eat?*; combining your chosen foods properly; proportioning those combinations well; speeding up your metabolism and slowing down your life. The last chapter in the section lays out the actual Diet Code program, which leads you through a three-part plan modeled on the path of classical tradespeople—from Apprentice to Journeyman to Master—with varied intensity according to your abilities and desires. There's a gentle initiation for beginners, including the specific formula for creating Diet Code meals, more specifics and details in a more intense phase in the middle of the learning curve, and a final phase in which you can relax into a lifetime of eating according to the program, having internalized the principles and reached your ideal weight.

Finally, in part III, I share advice on creating and maintaining a Diet Code kitchen, a range of flexible meal plans, and delicious, proportionally balanced recipes that are as quick to make as they are delectable. Diet Code food is inspired by the tastes and smells of my grandmother's Italian kitchen, honed by the ancient numbers of the Golden Ratio and presented here to allow you to get dinner ready in half an hour or less while stabilizing your weight and health without experiencing even a day of deprivation.

This book is a blend of ancient lore, Renaissance history, higher mathematics, hard science, personal stories, smart nutritional information and mouthwatering recipes anyone can manage. It unites the structural, mathematical principles of the cosmos that govern the growth of natural life and the aesthetic of natural beauty with wholesome, Mediterranean foods in a breakthrough formula for health, vitality and weight control. It's a provocative yet practical system of nutrition based on an intriguing mathematical phenomenon that's been utilized for millennia but never before applied to nourishing the human body. That makes this book absolutely unique in offering a more sustainable approach to food and eating pegged not to eliminating any one food group but to eating for enjoyment and pleasure, promoting health and reaching an ideal weight. My passion for excellent food, together with my understanding of how to combine the right foods for health, satisfaction and weight loss, gives you a plan you can quickly and easily put to work in your own life in your own kitchen, rediscovering along the way your natural waistline as well as the pure joy of eating for pleasure.

Our rightful heritage of wholesome eating as embodied by Leonardo's daily fare has been lost amidst our modern culture of fast food, fad diets and food phobias. The last three decades in particular, dominated by low-fat and then low-carb regimes that ensured nothing more than hordes of Americans eating in disastrously unnatural and imbalanced ways, have left us in sorry shape physically (more than 65% of Americans are overweight or obese) and even spiritually. Experts have calculated that obesity now cuts more years off our life spans than does cancer or heart disease. Americans have dieted furiously, yet grown ever fatter, no matter which way the prevailing dietary winds blow. It is time to dump the diets that have not just failed us but also aggravated (and even created) the obesity problem in favor of a lifestyle plan that will really work, once and for all. It is a lifestyle plan that puts an end to fad diets, a lifestyle plan from the ages, for the ages. The Diet Code reflects an ancient way of eating we've fallen away from. It's rightfully ours, however, and we need to reclaim it.

CHAPTER TWO

Discovering the Diet Code

The Ancients, having taken into consideration . . . the human body, elaborated all their works . . . according to these proportions.
—LUCA PACIOLI, DE DIVINA PROPORTIONE, 1509

When the ancients discovered Phi, they were certain they had stumbled across God's building block for the world . . .
—DAN BROWN, THE DA VINCI CODE

My personal journey to the place where the Golden Ratio and food and nutrition came together for me now seems as inevitable as the numbers themselves. Graham Green wrote, "There is always a moment in childhood where the door opens and lets the future in." Such a door swung wide for me a long time ago, and looking back, I observe the presence of the Golden Ratio even in my earliest years.

This is in spite of the fact that I was never much for math. C+ on report cards marked my best efforts. I *did* love bleaching and assembling animal skeletons, which I now see as representations of Golden Ratio math in action. Leonardo illegally exhumed cadavers to discover the precise Golden Ratio as present in the human body, and my early forays into anatomy prefigured a similar infatuation with ancient, sacred geometry.

Throughout my childhood I also spent untold hours tinkering in my grandfather's workshop. I can still clearly conjure the scene: Stanley hand planes, Buck Bros. chisels and drawknives, each wrapped in oiled canvas and cradled in a nested set of split oak oblong baskets he crafted himself. Just like those Russian Matryoshka dolls that stack within each other, the empty baskets would fit neatly one inside the next—an old-time tradesman's link to the Golden Ratio. The small basket is to the next larger basket as the larger basket is to the whole (the measure of both baskets).

The Golden Ratio, like that embodied by the baskets, sustains and replicates relationships in two directions at once. Any unit in the series creates the same relationship it has with the unit before it as with the unit after it. Any basket suggests the basket embracing it as well as the one it embraces. Any generation is simultaneously linked to its ancestry and its descendants.

The Diet Code is like that, too. The program combines the wisdom of the ancients and the science and art of the Renaissance with the traditions of my birth family, the needs of my own children and the demands of today's world into a diet and lifestyle plan that promises optimal health and easy weight loss.

In doing so, The Diet Code draws on the same ancient mathematical secrets that can take credit for at least some of the fascination with best-selling book *The Da Vinci Code,* which deals in part with the ramifications of the Golden Ratio in the work of Leonardo. Other great geniuses of the Renaissance employed it as well, as have legions of artists, architects, philosophers, mathematicians and scientists before and since. Our world is brimming with representations of the Golden Ratio, both naturally occurring and human-made; you'll see them yourself once you know what you're looking for.

In this chapter, I'll explain more about the math and history behind the Golden Ratio and trace my own path to discovering how its secrets could be applied to food and nutrition. Like the revelations uncovered in the novel *The Da Vinci Code,* this was a secret hiding in plain sight. I just had to learn how to see it.

THE GOLDEN RATIO

Before I lose any of you to math phobia, remember: This is someone with a grade-school C average in the subject talking. Just bear with me through the numbers, which I'll make as simple as possible, and keep in mind that when it comes to actually following The Diet Code program, the practice is much simpler than the theory. (Those of you who, on the other hand, wish to delve deeper into the math and history of the Golden Ratio should check out appendix B at the back of the book.)

The Golden Ratio, which governs the structure of our bodies as well as the structure of the universe, is a proportion related to a series of numbers now known as the Fibonacci sequence (1, 1, 2, 3, 5, 8, 13, 21, 34, 55, 89 . . .). In the Fibonacci sequence, each number is the sum of the previous two: $1 + 1 = 2, 1 + 2 = 3, 2 + 3 = 5, 3 + 5 = 8, 5 + 8 = 13$ . . . you get the idea. This series holds many fascinating numerical properties. What's important to us here is that any number in the series, divided by the number just before it in the series, gives nearly the same answer every time: 34 divided by 21 is 1.6190, and 55 divided by 34 is 1.6176, and 89 divided by 55 is 1.6181. As the series grows and the numbers get larger (144, 233, 337 . . .), the variance in those relationships, or ratios, gets smaller, hovering closer and closer to 1.618— a value also known as phi (pronounced "fee").

Phi is not an exact number; it is infinite. Beyond 1.618, it goes on forever without repeating any numbers pattern, no matter how many places you carry the decimal. Mathematicians call numbers like this *irrational*. This particular irrational number, revealed through ratios, is another way of expressing the Golden Ratio. Phi and other irrational numbers have proven to be very important in design: They create the formulae for curves.

The natural world is an astonishing display case of applications of phi, or the Golden Ratio. Phi first describes curves and spirals and then growth and movement. It can be found everywhere from a snail's shell or ram's horns to the arrangement of vertebrate skeletons and tree branches; it patterns the flight of birds and the swim courses of fish; the form of ocean waves and the shape and spin of galaxies. Another famous Italian, Galileo, got it right: The universe really is written in the language of mathematics. Plenty of examples of phi are also found throughout the human body—in the placement of joints, the development of the fetus, and the design of our kidneys, circulatory system and cerebrum.

The Golden Ratio keeps showing up because it works and works well. It's a proportion that guarantees efficient, economic and beautiful design. Great artists and architects throughout history have imitated and reiterated it, and musicians, geometers and scientists, among others, have used it to guide their work. In doing the same, Leonardo was in vast company.

In exploring the Golden Ratio, Leonardo essentially applied ancient wisdom, revivifying ideas older than ancient Greek or Egyptian civilization. What he observed and intuited in the world around him he presented in his art and other work. He matched his created patterns with universal design. What appeals to us so mightily, whether in the *Mona Lisa*'s smile, the interlaced façade of the Notre Dame, the curves of a Stradivari violin, the Great Pyramid—or even, as you'll soon see, a properly assembled plate of food—is the *rightness* of the design. We sense it reflects the correct order of things—an experience of what the world is, the reality of our own bodies—whether we're conscious of those connections or not. All of us are subconsciously in tune with the inherent design of the universe and recognize such beauty when faced with a reflection of that natural law. From each expression of the Golden Ratio, we get a sense of recognition: We are in a way looking at ourselves.

Now this proportion forms the foundation of the diet most closely aligned with the design of the human body, a diet designed in the same way as your body—a diet as efficient and effective as it is beautiful. That's what The Diet Code is all about: eating the way we are built to eat.

HOW LONG HAS THIS BEEN GOING ON?

In 1202, Leonardo ser Bonacci Pisano introduced to Western Europe couplets borrowed from Arabic and Vedic systems of math and poetry in which the next number in the sequence is determined by adding the two that come before it. This series became known as the Fibonacci (son of Bonacci) sequence.

The Golden Ratio is a proportion related to the Fibonacci sequence. "Golden Ratio" is a relatively new term for it. "Divine Proportion" was an earlier name first presented by Pacioli (a mathematician who followed the work of Fibonacci) in his fifteenth-century book of geometry—a book illustrated by none other than Leonardo da Vinci. "Golden Proportion" did not appear as a descriptive until the nineteenth century. Mathematicians generally agree, though, that phi was defined at least as early as 300 BCE by Euclid of Alexandria, of the Pythagorean school.

Legend has it that the Golden Ratio preceded even the Greeks, however, showing itself on the desert plains of Africa in ancient formulations for bread, alchemy and the shapes of pyramids. Back further still, Mesopotamian cultures, with their roots in the Carpathian Mountain and Black Sea regions, used sacred numbers and writings indicative of the Golden Ratio. Elaborate cave paintings of animals stylized with logarithmic curves dating to 15,000 years ago hint at an even more distant past. Whenever phi was first calculated, human beings have been immersed in its influence since we awakened to aesthetics some 35,000 years ago, even if it took many thousands of years more for us to be able to identify and use it. The story carrying the Golden Ratio and phi to you today is ancient, pointing toward universal truths humans have recognized essentially since they've left conscious record of themselves.

FROM WOODWORKER TO BAKER

I first used phi to perfect hand tools for woodworking. Dedicated to crafting by traditional methods, I quickly learned the importance of a properly shaped tool to getting the job done, getting it done well—and getting it done without wearing out my body. Looking for maximum efficiency, whether in a knife, a chisel or a saw handle, I found that making designs according to phi yielded just the right angles and curves. Form both preceded and followed function. The geometry of phi first displayed itself practically, in tools designed to fit the body. But it extended into the aesthetics of the tools; they were themselves a kind of everyday sculpture.

Our sense of beauty is attuned to nature and conditioned by the forms found there. We can recognize a pattern even without consciously knowing it and find that same great beauty in invented objects as well as in natural phenomena. As I later discovered, we can recognize that beauty in what we eat as well.

When I first moved to Maine, I struck up an informal arrangement with my neighbor Stan Joseph, exchanging woodworking lessons for meals. I'd teach him how to use a drawknife and shaving horse, tools dating back to ancient Egypt, and he'd fuel the exertion. One winter day after a long afternoon working in his barn, out came some aged cheddar, homemade hard apple cider, and rye bread he'd made himself. Resting in front of the fire crackling in the wood stove, satisfied with the work done, watching the sunset and enjoying the company, I swear it was the best thing I'd ever eaten. *What is this bread?* I thought to myself. *It tastes like life.*

Stan and I made a new deal: woodworking lessons for bread making lessons. His recipe started with a sourdough base of hand-milled rye berries and was baked for a long time at a low temperature, much like the bread made in ancient Egypt. I eagerly tried it on my own and, within about a month, Stan declared me twice the baker he could ever be. "This is your calling," he told me.

I soon wondered about the power of proportion in baking bread.

One of the main tricks to making good bread is figuring out how much water to add to a given amount of grain. The other is how much salt. All bakers have to confront these issues, and to find my own answers I turned to phi. The first loaves I made under its guidance were as vital as Stan's, but somehow lighter—springy and chewy without being gummy or heavy. Over the years since then, patrons have often raved about the almost mystical quality of my bread, and I'm convinced it's because my loaves follow this "Divine Proportion."

In bread baking, salt is used primarily to enhance the taste and strengthen the dough. When it comes to taste, our preference for salted bread is only about 200 years old; medieval and ancient loaves were rarely salted. Today, however, modern palates find unsalted bread to be somewhat insipid. In Tuscany, home of Leonardo and the purest "root cuisine" of Italy, the *pane* contains less salt than Americans are used to, and many of my customers come home from vacations there disappointed with it.

The Italian in me knows, however, that less salt yields a clean taste that is often a better foil for the simplicity of Italian cuisine. Still, my bread has to satisfy American appetites. Phi affords a perfect compromise: 1.618% salt (by weight, compared to flour) creates bread that matches what my customers crave while staying true to my ideas about good bread. In comparison, typical modern loaves have 2–2.5% salt—one and a half times as much.

I still sell in my bakery versions of the bread I learned to make from Stan all those years ago. The customer favorite is called *mattone* ("brick bread"). Even people allergic to wheat can enjoy it, since it is made with ancient unhybridized spelt, which is easier for the body to assimilate, and sourdough, which begins breaking down the grain, making it easier still for the body to handle. I make three more variations on Stan's original theme: *integrale,* "whole or complete bread," which, with sprouted lentils, millet and barley, is a complete vegetarian protein; *nero,* a "black bread" of crushed rye grains and rare black caraway; and *di giro,* "travel bread," a meal in itself incorporating mixed fruits and nuts, which I developed for the Maine Kayak Society.

I call them *abitare,* or breads of life.

THE GOLDEN PROPORTION OVEN

At the time I was refining my bread recipes, I lived in a small community of back-to-the-land pioneers in northern Maine that held a weekly potluck featuring fantastic produce from members' gardens, handcrafted cheeses, beers and wines, and seasonal fruit desserts. There was just one thing missing: bread. So that became my humble contribution. My skills as a baker developed quickly, and soon I was also bartering my bread for produce. I constructed a wood-fired stone oven in which to bake my bread. A word-of-mouth reputation soon had strangers searching out my bread.

When demand outgrew what I could bake in my own small oven, which could handle only six loaves at a time, I contracted with a local general store to use its pizza oven after closing. I'd mix up all the dough at my cabin in 5-gallon plastic buckets, drive it 40 minutes to the next town and stay up all night creating 100 or so loaves, experimenting with water and salt content to slow dough fermentation during those all-nighters. The whole process required a crazy system of scaffolding and wood planks winding through the tiny place to provide the multilevel structure I needed to raise and cool the bread, which, of course, I set up and broke down every single night.

I started selling loaves in other towns, and when demand once again outstripped my setup, I converted an old barn behind that general store into my first real bakery and built a 7-ton brick oven. I designed and built it according to the same proportions I had used in my woodworking and my bread recipes, carefully relating the depth of the deck of the hearth to the height of the ceiling, and so on. It was a huge investment, a crazy design, and I was no mason. But that oven would bake for 12 hours off one firing, on par with the best in this country. I baked up to 60 loaves at a time, maybe 300 loaves a day, in over 60 varieties throughout a year's seasonal rotation. Those breads were extraordinary, if I do say so myself, and I credit the Golden Proportion for successfully creating the dough and the oven that made it into bread.

I still make top-notch bread, thanks to the knowledge I've accumulated and the practice I've had in applying that knowledge. But back then, I owed it all to great ingredients and a great Golden oven.

FORMULATING THE DIET CODE

It wasn't until the Golden Proportion came into public consciousness with the enormous popularity of Dan Brown's *The Da Vinci Code* that I started to advertise the fact that I had been making bread according to its dictates for more than 20 years. By this time, I was based in a new bakery in Portland, Maine, named after the Greek word for wisdom: Sophia's. Bread and baked goods sales at Sophia's had been flagging in the midst of a national obsession with low-carb living, but people responded right away to the idea that bread like mine was perfectly in tune with the innate needs of the body.

More than just trying to sell bread, however, I was determined to sell people on a balanced lifestyle. I expanded my bakery into a café and began to apply the Golden Ratio to meals, too. I designed a line of "Da Vinci Plates," full meals that extended the properties of phi beyond baking into broader nutritional principles, balancing the major nutrients against each other in the Golden Ratio, just as I had done with bread dough ingredients. And I gave a series of lectures on my Leonardo-style diet plan.

I'd already developed a diet strategy for myself as part of my own quest to discover what to eat to keep my body at its best. I'd been interested in anatomy and physiology ever since I was a little kid and had studied microbiology and biochemistry in college. Cooking and nutrition connected those areas for me, and I had long dabbled in diet science, just for my own personal health. I researched calories, nutrients and metabolism. I made a study of different diets, reading up on them, comparing their requirements and recommendations and trying them out to see how I personally fared on them.

Experimentally, I'd varied my weight by almost 60 pounds, paring back to an ultra-lean 138 pounds on a strict carb-rich vegan regimen with lots of fruit, nuts and flat breads, and really bulking up, Rocky-style, swallowing raw eggs and drinking 2 gallons of milk a day until I tipped the scales robustly at nearly 200 pounds. In the process, I discovered that I was really comfortable in between, at 160 to 165 pounds on my 5-foot, 10-inch frame. That was where I really felt good about—and in—my body.

Aside from sizing up what worked for me, I'd never done anything to formalize the way I ate mathematically. I had a hunch that the same formulae that structure the universe—the same math that describes the human body—would naturally dictate a diet that would provide everything the body needed (and nothing it didn't) to fuel it throughout the day and throughout life. When I finally did do the math, linking carbohydrates, protein and fat together by exponents of phi, I realized that the proportions dictated by the Golden Ratio matched almost exactly the proportions I was eating already. In other words, the Golden Ratio created a diet I already knew first-hand—after years of personal experimentation—was ideal for me, my weight and my health. Numbers being a universal language, I had every reason to believe they'd hold the same promise for everyone. And, as it turned out, I was right.

The dietary percentages I derived through the Golden Ratio—the heart of The Diet Code—come to 52% of your calories from carbs (including vegetables and fruits as well as grains), 28% from fat and 20% from protein. While the math behind this is finicky, as those of you who venture into the "Do the Math" section are about to see, let me assure you that putting it into practice doesn't require such carefully calibrated precision. Feel free to make the translation into roughly one-half carb, one-third fat and one-fifth protein, as described more thoroughly below and in the Apprentice phase of the program in chapter 7. Creating the Golden Ratio on your plate, you see, is as easy as 1, 2, 3—when you think of it by weight rather than by calories: one part grain carbohydrate, two parts protein (in which category you're bound to find natural fat content) and three parts vegetables. (Remember that 1, 2, 3 and 5 are part of the Fibonacci sequence.)

DO THE MATH

Here I'm going to share how I worked out The Diet Code percentages with a series of simple equations, for those of you interested in the math. Follow along for the derivation of The Diet Code proportions, but if your eyes glaze over at mathematical notations, you can skip this box without missing anything important about to how to *apply* The Diet Code. So here goes:

The Diet Code balances macronutrients according to the Golden Ratio (measured by weight), such that

Fat × Phi (Φ) = Protein,
Protein × Φ^2 = Carb, and
Fat × Φ^3 = Carb.

Put another way, that's about 1.5 times as much protein as fat, 2.5 times as many carbs as protein and about 4 times as many carbs as fat.

To fill a hypothetical plate, you could begin with the following ratio:

10 grams of fat, which has 90 calories, since there are 9 calories per gram of fat. That would ideally be accompanied by
16.18 grams of protein (10 g fat × Φ), which has 64.72 calories, since there are 4 calories per gram of protein, and
42.36 grams of carbs (16.18 g protein × Φ^2), which has 169.44 calories, since there are 4 calories per gram of carb (10 g fat × Φ^3 concurs).

All together, that's a total of 324.16 calories in this meal. This, in turn, yields percentages in terms of calorie count:

90 out of 324.16 calories is 0.2776, or **28% fat**;
64.72 out of 324.16 calories is 0.1996, or **20% protein**;
169.44 out of 324.16 calories is 0.5227, or **52% carb**.

PUTTING IT TOGETHER

I was more or less hedging my bets with all this number crunching, when I was pretty sure what the outcome was going to be. I was confident that the same proportion that had worked everywhere else in my life, shaping my woodworking, baking and painting in particular, could be used to create a diet plan that optimized nutritional content and maximized weight loss. In fact, once I'd figured it all out and saw how it worked, I could have kicked myself in the head. *Why hadn't I thought of this before?*

The first day I started out to make a Golden meal, I meant to do it without ever compromising the principles of eating well I learned from my grandparents or the aesthetic principles I valued in other areas of my life.

The experiment began with scaling the weight of some slices of my bread. I'd been weighing pasta portions at home for years, wary of the inordinate helpings on the typical American plate, but I'd never thought to weigh a single-serving–size piece of my bread before. Next, in search of a protein, I found I had a simple tuna salad, made with lemon juice and olive oil (see recipe on p. 301), already in the fridge. I took the bread off the scale and measured out twice as much fish. Because tuna is extremely low in fat, I calculated in some olives to ensure a rough balance of fat and protein. To fill out the carb portion with vegetables (which is really what the American diet lacks), I added a portion of the cabbage salad my kids adore. I measured out a serving of that about three times the weight of the bread. Arranged all together on a plate, it looked very appealing. In fact, it also looked pretty much like what I served at home for supper.

From this one prototype, I created several variations to serve in the bakery café, focusing in every case on the most nutrient-dense foods I knew—high-quality fish, beans, olives, Italian greens, whole grain bread and so on (more on these Fundamental Foods in chapter 5). I had to consider the particular constraints of commercial cooking and serving food in what was originally set up specifically as a bakery. I had to keep in mind what was simple enough to prepare in a small, basic kitchen under the pressure of a lunch rush hour, easy enough to teach others to make, sturdy enough to keep well, tasty enough to appeal to a variety of palates, and elegant enough to satisfy my own and Sophia's standards. I needed dishes that minimized prep work and were quick to make and serve using readily available ingredients, besides being highly nutritious and, of course, delicious.

The first choices were very straightforward. These parameters streamlined my choices. Bread was a no-brainer—this was my bakery, after all—and for variety I added another Italian staple, polenta, as a major source of carbs. The protein choices were simple: cheese, white tuna, smoked herring, precooked organic sausage, eggs or grilled tempeh, prepared with a minimum of fuss. Any lean protein I simply bolstered with a little fat from olives or olive oil. The vegetables physically dominated the plate, so they needed to make more of a statement and were therefore more of a challenge. I finally settled on four basic approaches that met all my criteria: the cabbage salad I began with (see recipe on p. 278), braised greens (see recipe on p. 285), caponata (eggplant salad; see recipe on p. 258), and oven-roasted sweet peppers in tomato sauce (usually to accompany the sausage).

I was putting together meals much like my Italian grandparents would have enjoyed (simple, Italian peasant meals)—meals not much different from those that might have been served at a table in Tuscany, circa 1500. I soon had a half a dozen combinations I liked, which I called Da Vinci Plates—after Leonardo, of course—in honor of their revival of math and foods from five centuries ago.

I added these Da Vinci Plates to the Sophia's menu the next working day. Customer response was immediate and enthusiastic. The Da Vinci Plates quickly became, and remain, the most popular meals I sell. Despite the math or, more accurately, as a result of it, there's a naturalness to this food that increases its appeal and keeps patrons returning day after day.

Obvious indicators I was doing something right included the number of plates I served and the amount of food remaining on those

plates (none!) when customers left the shop. Also noticeable, however, was the fact that no one ever asked for more than what was
served, not even for another slice of bread or a few more olives. Although the proportions of these meals are different from what most
Americans are used to—at least those Americans used to the typical
sandwich lunch, featuring spongy white bread, a large amount of
meat and cheese, and very little vegetable, perhaps a slice of hothouse tomato or a leaf of nothing lettuce—I was offering basically
the same components (bread, protein, vegetable) but in radically different and in much more nourishing proportions. People really
responded to this more natural way to eat.

My customers find every satisfaction in these meals. The first rave
is always about the taste. Then I hear about how sustaining the food
is. Many people have told me that after a Sophia's lunch, they don't
need their usual afternoon pick-me-up. (Do I have to mention that's
usually a cookie or candy bar or some other junk food?) It is, after all,
about a pound of food altogether, and food dense with fiber as well as
nutrients at that. Just as your body knows it is hungry, it knows what
it is really hungry for. When you provide it with nutritious food, it has
what it needs in terms of fuel and nutrients, so it stops sending out
hunger signals. You end up eating less. The selections and combinations on a Da Vinci Plate also provide variety, so although I'm not
plating up the jumbo meals that are most restaurants' stock-in-trade,
my customers often comment that the meals are "just perfect."

Another constant comment is that these Da Vinci Plates *look* really
good. A lot sell by sight: one look at someone else's order, and a customer will stop me to ask what it is, then usually order the same.
Visual appeal comes from fresh ingredients and is heightened by
interesting sizes, shapes, colors and textures to catch the eye. Besides
that, the meals just look healthy and like the right amount of food
(neither too little nor too much). I think there's something else at
work, though—a natural human response to any observation of the
Golden Ratio. We recognize it when we see it and it resonates with
us, even if the medium is nothing more than a plate of food.

I also began to get feedback about how good people felt after eating this food, healthier and stronger. People started to ask about my secret, wanting to replicate the experience with what they prepared at home. Then I began to hear reports of weight loss, and I knew I was really on to something. I'd cracked The Diet Code!

I'd already experienced for myself what a difference eating this way could make. While I remodeled the space that became Sophia's, I worked long days and couldn't cook for myself, and so I was eating out a lot. I was grabbing sandwiches, sodas and the like—whatever I could grab and eat in a hurry. It didn't take me long to pack on about 15 extra pounds. In my late 30s, I was a victim of the dreaded "middle-age spread."

But that excess weight dropped right off when I consciously followed a Mediterranean-style diet—when the shop finally opened, life settled down (a little!) and I went back to preparing most of my own meals. Then, when I developed (and adopted) The Diet Code plan, with properly proportioned meals, I got noticeably leaner and more muscular. As my metabolism increased, the flabby fleshiness I still had from my Year of Eating Dangerously vanished. On The Diet Code program, my weight has stabilized, even though now I'm well into my 40s, at about 162 pounds (which appeals to me additionally as a representation of phi).

So I was already clear on the fact that this diet was right for me. But once I saw my benefits replicated in others, I knew this was something I had to share. Using the foods and math that created the Da Vinci Plates, expanding the options to include breakfast, dinner and snacks (Sophia's Da Vinci Plates are essentially a lunch trade) as well as compatible lifestyle choices beyond food (but equally important to true nourishment), I designed a flexible, comprehensive program meant to be used at home, every day, by absolutely anyone who's ready to end the battle of the bulge once and for all. Your journey is about to begin.

Chapter Three

We Are What We Eat

Do not seek the way of the ancients; seek what they sought.
—Bashō

*Bread [has] a whole mythology which speaks of wisdom,
patience, mysterious goodness and technological expertise.*
—Margaret Visser, from *Much Depends on Dinner*

I come from a mixed family: dark rye on one side, *pagnotta* on the other. My mom's family bought huge sections of black rye flavored with pungent black caraway from Turkestan, baked in behemoth loaves at a family-owned shop in Colchester, Connecticut, that still might as well have been in Poland. My dad's family bought Italian bread imported all the way from New Jersey. A thick, brittle crust that splintered into shards and tasted of caramel shielded a transparent crumb that was open-celled and sturdy as honeycomb.

The rye was a meal with smoked herring or ham and a side of sauerkraut. Papa Mazurkiewicz liked it best smeared with bacon grease, tiled with sliced radish or onion, and coarsely salted. The pagnotta was a meal as an edible spoon dipped into tomato sauce, with a small side plate of cold boiled chicken. An after-school snack at Nona Louisa's was bread, olive oil, homemade vinegar peppers and very sharp provolone, broken up almost like little quarried blocks of Cararra marble. Either way, one taste and you knew you were home.

Food says a lot about who we are. Cultures and peoples define themselves in part by what they eat and how they eat it. The choice, preparation and sharing of food not only reflects the climate and geography of a place but also shapes the society elementally. Sharing food and meals bonds people as an important cultural and societal glue.

Currently, what our food is saying about us, as Americans, is not good. We're industrialized (dehumanized), denatured, chemically enhanced, fake and always focused on speed over nutrition, profit over sustainability and quantity over quality. I don't know about you, but that's definitely not who I want to be.

There is a better way, but we've fallen drastically out of touch with it. Nutritionally dense foods eaten in natural proportions once sustained human society, but we've abandoned them. It's like there was a golden age in the past, and we are the poorer for having lost it. That's especially sad, because by rights, *this* should be our golden age. We have access to more than ever, both materially and in terms of ideas and wisdom. Those who came before us didn't have all the resources, information and technology we have today, yet they had the wisdom to eat in tune with the body. We've advanced so much in some ways, but in others we've lost a lot of ground. The Diet Code is a way to tune back into what we never should have let go.

In our solely American framing of food not as nourishment but as mechanism—with its dark rumbling of food fears and anxieties—we have turned our backs on the poetic wisdom of the ancients. Most recently this has taken the form of carb-phobia, so the most urgent message we need to hear is *Grain is good*. But that's just the beginning. The greater theme of balance, as determined by the Golden Ratio and now applied to particulars in The Diet Code, frees us to enjoy our food as well as receive all its benefits.

Part of what's happened in our fast, prepackaged food culture is that we are no longer intimately familiar with what we eat—where it comes from, how it is made and what it is like in its natural state. Preparing your own food is one of the best ways to easily follow The Diet Code and to get back in touch with what you eat. That's the way to free yourself from the strictured, fearful ways in which Americans so often approach food and eating and begin connecting with the pleasure and satisfaction of good food that is well prepared.

We act as if we no longer have time to sit down and enjoy a meal, as if we don't remember how to savor what we eat—or as if doing those things is something reserved for special occasions spent eating in high-end restaurants. But these are skills we need to hone every day, in our homes, whether the food before us is simple or sophisticated. Start with real food—good food. When we're eating commercially prepared foods, which don't really taste that good or, at least, that interesting, it's no wonder we wolf them down. But when we do that, we end up either still eating long after we are really full (but having not yet received the "enough" signal from the body) or eating on mindlessly in a futile attempt to get what the body really needs (but will never get from junk food). Real food, like what's recommended on The Diet Code, has more flavor and more sophisticated fragrances, which get us excited about what we are eating. Real food also takes longer to eat. It spends longer in the mouth, which ultimately improves digestion and absorption of nutrients, and we spend longer at the table eating a smaller amount of food (calorically speaking). We then have plenty of time to notice when our bodies are telling us they have had enough. After all, food is just one part of the best meals. The other is the company. With real food on the table, we'll have plenty of time to enjoy both.

My livelihood gives me a particular window onto the value of what's largely gone missing between us and what we eat, as well as a view of what happens when we experience remembering. The physical act of making bread is a connection with history. The process awakened in me an awareness of the cultural histories each loaf represented—the family hearth and shared meals it evoked. It's a large part of why I choose to do what I do; there's no arguing with the physical authenticity of kneading great mounds of dough by hand, as has been done for centuries. And there's no arguing with the satisfaction of making something so primal, so ancient, so nourishing and so nurturing—and then sharing it with others. The process of cooking for yourself, at least some of the time, can provide you with an experience similar to the one I experience when making bread.

—⚉—

To help you understand the importance of reclaiming the physical and emotional connection to our food, I will trace the history of a particular food to show you what it has meant to us—and thereby what we're missing when we disrespect that heritage. I could pick

---

TALKING ABOUT BREAD

From "bread-and-butter" issues to "breaking bread together," language reflects just how important and ingrained loaves are in human life and culture. For instance, something highly valued costs a lot of "bread" or "dough." And think about these:

"Bread is the staff of life."
"The best thing since sliced bread."
"Give us this day our daily bread."
"Know which side your bread is buttered on."

And while we talk a lot about bread in English, listen to what they say in Italian (with thanks to *The Italian Baker* by Carol Field):

Buono come il pane ("As good as bread"; used to refer to someone or something you can really count on; down to earth and good-hearted)

Trovar pane per i propri denti ("To find bread for one's teeth"; to meet your match)

Dire pane al pane e vino al vino ("To call bread, bread and wine, wine"; or, as Americans put it, "To call a spade a spade")

Essere pan e cacio ("To be like bread and cheese"; to be natural companions)

from many examples—wine, or olive oil, or rice and beans—and reveal through them short histories of the human condition. But I'm a baker, so I chose bread.

Bread embodies both personal and cultural memories. Just a whiff of fresh bread can easily transport you to particular times and places in your own life. Likewise, whole cultures define themselves by their bread: tortilla, biscuit, pita, nan, vollkornbrot, baguette, focaccia, matzoh, johnnycake, injera and so on. Bread is a hallmark of a people. At the epicenter of any community, with the same pride of place as a house of worship, there will be a bakery. Take away the bread, and the center will not hold.

The author Susan Seligson writes about the passion incited by this "simple union of flour, water and salt" in *Going with the Grain: A Wandering Bread Lover Takes a Bite Out of Life*. "People will suffer any number of indignities, but triple the price of bread and whether it is contemporary Jordan or 18th century France, they take to the streets in angry hordes." Throughout the ages, she points out, bread has fired political protests, inspired poets and been pressed into service by religions around the world. The Italians have a proverb: *Senza il pane tutti divento orfano*—loosely translated, "Without bread, everyone is an orphan." The Arabs go further, denoting both bread and life with a single term: *aysh*.

Bread is a component of our physical and spiritual development. Seligson continues, "Now bread is being relegated to the . . . list of so-called 'bad' foods. This is a terrible shame and a notion that would be met by stunned disbelief in most parts of the world. . . . When you demonize bread, you demean life itself." I'd argue we don't even have to demonize bread to achieve that end: we do it just the same when we accept highly processed, nonnutritious factory-made versions of it (or any food), snapping the connection to the history and mystery of the real thing.

Bread has been considered sacred in many times and places and can be one of the most important things we eat. We can't live by bread alone, of course, although in point of fact, I *do* make some breads that, nutritionally speaking, are a meal unto themselves. We need a wide variety of natural foods to sustain us. But I'm here to say, "Bread is back!" We've learned the hard way about the many flaws of excising a food group from our diets (carbs, say), wreaking imbalance on ourselves. Peak physical and mental condition requires a balance of macronutrients, including carbs. And so does a permanently trim waistline.

A BRIEF HISTORY

Our history and the history of our food are inextricably linked. We need to come to grips with both. If we don't know where we've come from, it's that much harder to see where we want to go. We've forgotten our past and, as far as diet goes, at least, are being condemned by *not* repeating it. The central notion of The Diet Code is to remember and reapply what we (collectively) once knew, the same way Leonardo caught hold of ancient math and utilized it in even the most forward-thinking of his projects. Here again, I'll use my baker's prerogative and take bread as my example.

Societies throughout history have been founded on grain- and carbohydrate-based diets much like the one touted in *The Diet Code*. Thousands of years after modern humans colonized the Black Sea region, bearing all-important language skills and advanced stone tools, climate change allowed for the appearance of primitive forms of wheat, such as einkorn and emmer. These grains spurred the beginnings of agricultural societies. Learning to cultivate the earth, plant seed and store grain as protection against lean times gave groups of people more stability and more predictable living conditions than ever before. Ensuring a steady food supply allowed for permanent settlements. This let civilization as we know it take root and develop. Humans who knew where their next meal was coming from could devote time to developing skills beyond hunting and gathering.

As people learned to raise a variety of grains and other crops and adapted to their particular regions, early forms of bread were developed. Agricultural techniques inevitably advanced in tandem with the societies that developed them. One advancement to note in particular is the crossing of emmer with an indigenous Persian grass to produce spelt, the first modern wheat.

Making grain into bread—one of the first known foods requiring real preparation—heralded another stage in cultural development. Even in Neolithic times, nomadic tribes mixed water with cereal grains they crushed with stones and cooked the resulting paste into flat cakes on hot stones over open fires. The earliest breads were like tortilla or chapati—thin, unleavened leaves of mixed grains, perhaps baked on mounds of hot sand. Cakes of wheat and barley parched in the desert sun have been found in Jericho dating to 8,000 years ago. Egyptians then developed a precursor to leavened bread, probably made from partially sprouted grains. The first raised breads were baked in Egypt in around 3000 BCE. (Excavations of ancient Egyptian tombs have revealed intact loaves baked over 5,000 years ago, which you can see today in the British Museum!)

Peoples around the planet have enjoyed bread ever since, each developing a signature bread based on the grains and methods best

---

BREAD AROUND THE WORLD

If we were to plot the evolution of bread across time and around the globe, tracing the varying kinds of dough, we'd see a geographic Fibonacci spiral emerge from the emanative center of Egypt. If you'll indulge a baker's technical knowledge for a moment: One of the definitive characteristics of any bread is the relation of water to flour used. Bread doughs generally become progressively drier as they evolve westerly and forward in time, moving from the poured batter *bedja* bread of Egypt to the unruly doughs of Turkey and Syria that bake up so ethereally, through the irregular loaves of Italy (often mixed too wet to need scoring), next the less hydrated formal breads of France and on to the dry biscuit and crumbly bairmbrack of the British Isles.

suited to their particular climate and geography. In this way, bread signifies both our unity and diversity: All our ancestors made bread, and all our ancestors made their own special kind of bread.

Bread furthered the development of cultures in specific and perhaps a bit surprising ways. Bread was assigned even greater importance than simple sustenance. Egyptians used loaves as currency; workers, including those who built the pyramids, were often paid in bread. Bread, provider of simple sustenance and so literally the stuff of life, was used to honor the gods—especially Osiris, the god of fertility.

THE FIVE SENSES

The prepackaged blandness of most grocery store sliced bread is a crime against history and nature—and the perfect symbol of the terrible disconnect between us and our relationship with whole food.

Properly done, bread making is a fully sensual, hands-on process. I gauge much of what I need to know about a batch of dough or a loaf of bread by the senses. I can tell by smell when the loaves are done. Bakers, like perfumers and vintners, develop quite a nose. I often run to the oven to pull down the door on my latest batch, alerted by the intoxicating rightness of a full-bodied, buttery, caramel odor, only to hear the timer go off behind me.

A really good loaf of bread visually sports at least four colors—from white to black, with displays of ruddy sienna and deep umber brown. Some breads craze, crackle and pop as they hit the cooler air outside the oven, creating little firework shards of crust that tell you your timing is right. Tap the bottom of a finished loaf, and you'll hear a specific tone: a hollow ring, confirming its readiness. These are my favorite moments in the process, pulling bread out of the oven, soaking in the subtle clues telling you you've done a good job.

Making bread this way is my way of standing strong in a fast-moving, technologically oriented, largely prefabricated culture, preserving local business in an era of multinational corporations. I moved four hours south of the town that housed my original wood-fired brick oven ten years ago and have since adapted to using standard gas-fired ovens that retain only the brick hearth. But the old process remains the same. It's no coincidence that my customers find more soulful satisfaction in a handmade loaf here than they do in a plastic-wrapped loaf from the supermarket. The same happens when we choose whole, fresh, real food of any kind. It's always better than prefabricated, overly processed or fake food. We know it, and our bodies know it. That's why tasting the real thing (no matter *what* we're eating) is one of the core themes of The Diet Code.

FOOD AS RITUAL

Food once nourished us physically but also psychologically, connecting us with our culture and our roots and providing us with ritual as well. And not just obvious rituals, like communion, seder or a Ramadan break-fast. Ritual is all about the connection we have to the things we do each day, over and over. Diet is a part of that. From the Latin word *dies* ("of a day") and the Greek word *diaitasthai* ("to lead one's life"), *diet* emerges as daily conduct or rite of life.

The Diet Code takes us back to a time before food became commerce. Fad diets are now all about big business and not about health. Trendy takes on weight loss became the rage through marketing and lobbying, not through touting superior nutrition. We even got sold on a scheme (low-carb) that works, to the extent it does, because it mimics starvation.

We need meals that we can look forward to. We can't all participate in the meaningful ritual of baking bread, but a diet that places bread and other foods of the ancients at its core sparks a mythos that can excite us each day. We say, "You are what you eat," but in more profound ways, food can tell us who we are, where we came from and where we are going.

Glenn O'Brien writes about something similar but in the context of fashion in "Requiem for a Tux" from *BlackBook* (January 2005): "Before fashion became commerce, clothing was cultural and ceremonial. It created form. Formality created form. People had good form or bad form. Good form connected people to their culture, to their roots, to the path of true social progress. . . . Black tie was ceremonial. The cocktail dress and . . . even the miniskirt, were ceremonial: fashion as an integral part of . . . cultural practice and ritual."

In concluding, O'Brien, too, makes the connection to food: "Perhaps there is still something magical in [ritual]. . . . When you get dressed, think about what it means. When you have a meal, do the same. Once, gods oversaw the little rituals, giving meaning to the smallest human actions, the ones we repeat endlessly. If we pay attention to what we're doing . . . , it might lead us back to culture, back to a life filled with the riches of meaning."

The Diet Code's focus on whole foods and a healthier lifestyle promises not only weight loss, but also a reconnection to the ritual of eating—and the magic and meaning of doing so.

Part II

FOLLOWING THE CODE

Chapter Four

Goodfellas and Fugazy: Whole Carbs, Whole Foods, and Why Fake Food Is Fattening

Human subtlety . . . will never devise an invention more beautiful, more simple or more direct than does nature, because in her inventions nothing is lacking, and nothing is superfluous.

—Leonardo da Vinci,
The Notebooks, Vol. I, ch. 1

Everything has been said before, but since nobody listens, we have to keep going back and beginning all over again.

—André Gide

"Come sta quelle cosa?"
"Che cosa . . . quelle cosa o l'altra cosa?"
We've heard it all before, phrased in some mob movie or on *The Sopranos*—classic Italian circular speaking:
"How's that thing?"
"What thing . . . that thing or the other thing?"
It's a comedic quandary. What's not so funny is finding out Americans have been doing essentially this—going around in circles—when it comes to the juggler's act of diets we have tossed about for the last four decades.

No fat. No eggs. No beef. No wheat. No carbs. Fad diets of simple exclusion work temporarily because they break habit and disrupt metabolism. But subtraction is the wrong math. With it, we just keep buying into new deficiencies.

As H. L. Mencken put it, "For every complex problem, there is a solution that is simple, neat and wrong." The human body—and its care and feeding—is complex to begin with, and furthermore varies from individual to individual. When we buy into oversimplification like this, we are not only doomed to failure and incurring risk but also missing the logic of an approach that embraces the whole. The medical community can't agree on any one plan that actually works, much less one that works for everyone.

Misguided fat-free promotions like the Stillman Diet and the Pritikin Eating Plan burdened Americans with excess refined carbs which in turn led us to carb-phobia. Clinging to ghastly egg white omelets, skinless poultry and nonfat dairy products, we suffered first the banishment of fat and now the rebound of blackballed carbs. We forked over top dollar for chemical cardboard and other joyless boxed industrifoods that never satisfied true hunger or need for nourishment.

The words *fad* and *fade* come from the Vulgar Latin *fatuus,* meaning vapid, vacuous, insipid or tasteless—just like a diet without carbs or fat. Fad diets are destined to fade, and yet we entrust our fate to them. Fad diets bent on eliminating a food group wholesale are imbalanced, unnatural, unhealthy, ineffective and even potentially lethal. They are also making us fatter. Even those espoused by doctors have drastically altered the proportions in which we eat the three macronutrients (carbohydrates, fat and protein) to an extent that is endangering our long-term health.

Modern medicine has failed us. We live without preventative health care or a sustainable health care system. Aside from serious accidental injury, most bodily afflictions, including obesity, arthritis, heart and lung ailments and even cancer, are directly related to diet. Yet doctors are poorly schooled in nutrition; their training focuses instead on the dispensation of drugs. No wonder their diet "revolutions" are characterized by a disregard for proportion. The inherent imbalance keeps us dependent on laboratory-born food additives, industrial food substitutes and often assorted pharmaceuticals. *Oobatz!* It's crazy, and it keeps us fat.

GIU DI FORMA

Carbs aren't what's making us fat. And fat didn't make us fat either. For that we can blame *giu di forma*—badly formed or unfit food. Blame processed junk. There's plenty of it. Cheap, fractured food is available everywhere we turn, around the clock—high-calorie beverages; snack and fast foods in outsized portions; low-fat this and low-carb that, packed with calories as well as artificial fat, sugar and carb substitutes. The majority of products ringing the outside of our grocery stores may be fit food *(in forma)*, but just about everything else in the vast middle acreage of aisles is processed, refined and artificially altered to within an inch of its life.

Leonardo would have been hard-pressed to recognize any of it as something humans could or should eat. Even if he wasn't familiar with tomatoes and potatoes (which didn't arrive in Europe from the New World until pretty near the end of his lifetime), he'd surely comprehend them at a basic level. But just imagine him trying to wrap his mind around fluorescent green ketchup or fries made of rehydrated potatoes extruded into smiley-face shapes.

Neither bread nor butter is inherently fattening. It isn't any one type of food that makes us fat; it is the panoply of foods terribly distorted from the way nature made them that does it. Yes, carbs and fats can cause problems: Refined sugars and starches and synthetic oils *do* have adverse health effects, but so do all other denatured macronutrients, like ultra-lean meats, fat-free dairy, margarine and hydrogenated fats, artificial sweeteners and synthetic mimics, like soy cheese and soy meats. In their natural forms, both carbs and fats are ideal nutrition for the human body.

Every time some fad diet hits the big time, however, our stores are flooded seemingly overnight with "new" foods tailored to the trend of the moment. As low-carb and low-fat became industries unto themselves, following these plans was no longer a matter of choosing from available natural foods that met the guidelines and were generally healthful. Suddenly, manufactured products were everywhere, including obvious logical inconsistencies, like low-carb candy, low-fat whipped cream, low-carb hamburger buns and nonfat potato chips and patently ridiculous advertising claims like those proclaiming low-carb water. Natural fiber got replaced with polydextrins and other indigestible starches, which proliferated as filler. Sugar replacements such as sorbitol, mannitol and glycerol—disguised carbohydrates all—filled low-carb products. Fried foods were dipped in indigestible fats—so indigestible that they caused unpleasant gastrointestinal side effects in many unwary consumers.

Not only were we being sold chemical "food," but also a bill of goods. Those artificial sweeteners and sugar alcohols impair the body's natural ability to sense caloric load and regulate appetite. The body doesn't recognize them as nutrients the way it does sugar, and they don't trigger the physiological signals that tell us we are full. In other words, we lose our natural ability to tell when we've had enough. We'll go on eating and craving more the more we eat, suggests a Purdue University study published in the *International Journal of Obesity*. "Diet" foods are actually making us fatter.

Beyond that, some of these artificial ingredients bind to fat and disrupt the normal process of metabolizing it. Some are carcinogenic over time. None has nutritional benefits or nutritional value; they are completely nonnutritive. (And then we end up being sold supplements to give us back the fiber, good fats, minerals and vitamins that have been stripped from the foods they rightfully belong in. Think of how crazy it is to buy wheat germ and wheat bran to go with a white-flour diet!) And they are, of course, chemicals not naturally found in the body, making them prime suspects for mischief. Some, like neurotoxic aspartame, are proven hit men.

In this chapter, I'll take you through some basic information about carbs and fats and their effects on the body, which will come in handy as you embrace The Diet Code and this new/old way of eating. I'll expose the flaws in the nutritional myths that have hobbled us for too long and put forth instead a guide created from a whole-body, whole-life perspective. Whole foods, the "goodfellas," are good for you; "fugazy," or fake versions, are not.

CHE BRUTA—HOW UGLY IT IS

Americans don't have a problem with carbs; they have a problem with "brute" versions nutritionally destroyed by overprocessing. Grains divested of most of their iron, fiber, B vitamins, antioxidants, trace minerals, phytochemicals, and even a good chunk of protein and fat in the germ are called "refined"—but this belies their heavy-handed way with the body. White flour is actually about 10% higher in calories because the good stuff has been taken out of it. And what's left is digested very quickly in the body—essentially the same as straight sugar—sending blood sugar levels to an unhealthy spike, resulting in a surge of insulin released from the pancreas to reduce it.

It's like a bar full of brutish drinkers that explodes into a riot. The bouncers (like insulin) rush the crowd out, but if the place empties completely, it's bad for business. So they want a new batch of patrons. Similarly, as your blood sugar is reduced, your body wants that quick burst of energy back—it feels hungry and craves more food, particularly more sugar. That's why it is so easy to overdo it once you get started with unhealthy carbs. The more of this junk you eat, the more of this junk you want to eat.

Run your body through this addictive cycle too many times, and you are on the pathway to insulin resistance in which, just as it sounds, your body becomes numb to the efforts of insulin. It becomes rougher, and takes longer, to get sugar out of your blood. And you are prediabetic.

The way to keep your risk of progressing to diabetes down is to stop overcrowding the house. Take a page from Leonardo, who observed the dangers of overpopulation as a major cause of the spread of the Black Death. He presented Sforza of Milan with a civic design for preventative health, proposing finite neighborhoods with adequate roadways, utilities and sanitation. His growth formula for a city is no different than the proper proportion of foods needed by the body.

To prevent frequent surges of insulin, you need to limit simple carbs and focus instead on eating a spread of beneficial whole carbs,

---

AN APPLE A DAY . . .

. . . provides an eighth of your daily requirement of fiber, yet contains significantly more carbs (25 grams) than you'd be allowed in the Induction phase of the Atkins Nutritional Approach. With that draconian attitude, the apple takes up an association with evil last encountered in the Garden of Eden.

It's absurd to routinely pass up something that's less than 100 calories, a good source of potassium, folic acid, vitamin C and other antioxidants, and juicy, sweet and crisp! It's no wonder apples are one of the world's most popular fruits and helps explain why there are some 7,500 varieties to choose from today.

The Romans established the first consistently cultivated varieties of apples (seven of them by the sixth century BCE) and created a deity of fruit trees, the goddess Pomona. They were working from a lineage reaching back to the wild apples that may have come from the forests of the Tien Shan Mountains in Kazakhstan. Apples were found among the early settlements of the Jordan River Valley (6500 BCE), and by 2500 BCE, the royalty of Ur in Mesopotamia favored the fruit. By the thirteenth century BCE, Ramses II had apple trees planted along the Nile Valley.

As for the association with sin, that fate didn't befall the apple until Leonardo's time. In 1470, Hugo van der Goes painted *The Fall of Man,* depicting the fruit of the tree of knowledge in the Garden of Eden as apples. Surely you aren't still holding arbitrary biblical symbolism against it!

fats and protein, all of which are more slowly digested, occasioning a slow and steady release of insulin that your body is equipped to handle gracefully.

The empty calories of overprocessed carbs carry little nutritional value, yet make up the bulk of the average American diet and help to make you fat and keep you that way. They also create the right breeding ground for your in-body plagues of anxiety, anemia, arthritis, osteoporosis, viral infection and cancer.

Overprocessed carbs wreak havoc with the hormonal balance of food metabolism and wrap you with a "spare tire." Bad carbs go straight to your belly, it seems. Researchers showed a strong association between the amount of highly refined grains in the diets of otherwise healthy men and women and the size of their waists in relation to their hips. The study demonstrated that the people who preferred refined grains increased by a whole pants size over the three-year span of the study. That was *three times* the rate of growth of participants who got the bulk of their carbs from whole grains, fruits and vegetables. Those whose diets were lower in fiber tended toward a balloon shape associated with increased risk of heart disease. Participants who got more fiber were more tapered in their silhouettes (even at similar weights)—like the ancient Egyptians pictured in temple artwork.

FUEL UP WITH CARBS

You crave carbs not because of some perverse joke of nature—longing for what's worst for you—but because your body *needs* them. Cutting out something as basic to normal body functioning as carbs defies common logic, not to mention physio-logic. You may as well eliminate water! Carbohydrates are your body's most efficient fuel source, so carbohydrate metabolism is your default setting for getting energy. Your body cleanly breaks down carbohydrates (starches and sugar) into the glucose it uses to power every cell it has. In contrast, the breakdown of protein for fuel leaves toxic ammonia, which,

INSULIN BUILDS MUSCLE

To maintain blood sugar in a specific health range (70–100 milligrams per deciliter), the pancreas pumps out insulin to bind to the glucose that comes from digesting carbs and store it as potential energy in the muscles and liver, and secondarily in fat cells. So insulin often gets blamed for making people fat. That's a bum rap, though. Insulin is an integral part of body mechanics and stores glucose as fat *only* in response to the overeating of refined carbs. The problem comes only when people throw off the balance of the system.

When the system is in balance, fueled by whole carb foods, insulin initiates the building of muscle and organ tissue (body proteins), not fat cells. On the other hand, if you are not exposed to enough insulin—if you are taking in too much protein or inadequate carbohydrates—glucagon, another endocrine hormone that works in concert with insulin, will be pressed into service in catabolic (breaking down) metabolism, essentially deconstructing muscle, liver and fat cells. Burning off fat this way may seem desirable, but the cost (burning off muscle as well) is far too high. It's far better to build muscle through both exercise and a carb-rich diet. Increased muscle mass raises your metabolism, which burns glucose—and fat stores—in a self-regulating cycle.

flushed out as urea, is dehydrating and can rob the body of minerals, especially calcium.

You need carbohydrates for the full functioning of both brain and brawn. Ninety percent of the glucose in your body serves the brain, and carbs are the preferred fuel for muscles under exertion. Carbs build and power muscles. Top-flight athletes cannot perform without carbs, and neither can you. This makes them the "big earners" of the diet—the largest part of your caloric intake should be from carbohydrates.

It should be no surprise that it's a *lack* of carbs that can be dangerous to your health, well-being and waistline. If you don't get enough carbs, muscle and brain functions actually slow down or even stop. Facing a dearth of carbs, your body will essentially digest its own muscle and organ tissues to get the fuel it needs.

Along with basic brain function, your mood may also be affected by low levels of carbohydrates. Cutting back too far on beneficial carbs can leave you with anxiety or depression, or even obsessive-compulsive behavior. Short of that, when your brain runs low on fuel, you might experience mild to moderate difficulty concentrating, mental fuzziness, sexual dysfunction, restlessness, irritability or a general sense of discontent. That's because your brain works optimally on full power, of course, and also because it needs the glucose from carbs to make serotonin, a neurotransmitter that lifts your mood and makes you feel calm. Serotonin also improves sleep and pain tolerance. The B vitamins, of which whole grain carbs are a rich source, are also necessary for making the neurotransmitters crucial to keeping your brain and your whole nervous system running smoothly. According to the American Dietetic Association, taking in low levels of B vitamins also makes it harder for you to handle stress. If you had your brain chemistry tested before and after eating carbs, you'd see increased serotonin levels within minutes.

Carbs, in short, make you feel good. It's no wonder you crave them especially when you are tired, upset or stressed. Doing without carbs when you need them this way never helps you, in the short or long term. You've probably felt it yourself if you've ever tried seriously restricting carbs. After a while—be it hours or weeks—you're bound to overdo it whenever you do finally give in. That yo-yo, from denial to overindulgence, is a hallmark of following a low-carb diet, and your human hardwiring is to blame. The cravings for carbs have a powerful physiological as well as psychological basis.

REMEMBRANCES OF DIETS PAST

In point of fact, the low-carb fad has already come and gone, but as people who have forgotten the past, we are condemned to repeat it. The low-carb Banting scheme, developed by the undertaker (!) William Banting, swept London in the 1860s. He indulged in an unbalanced diet of milk, refined bread, pastry, beer and meat that pushed his 5-foot, 6-inch frame to over 200 pounds.

Banting lost weight when he reduced carbs, removing sugar and dairy from his diet, thereby inventing the first modern fad diet. He lost about 5 pounds a month following a plan of three 4- to 6-ounce servings of meat or fish and three small servings of bread a day, along with the addition of vegetables. His solution to avoiding sugar cravings bolstered his carb intake, though: half a dozen glasses a day of fortified wine!

It's no coincidence that the first fad diet—the first perceived *need* for a fad diet—arose during the period of Industrial Revolution. Part of that Revolution was replacing the water- and wind-powered stone mills of the preceding 2,000 years with new steel roller mills. That made denatured flour widely available for the first time in history. Humans were quick to misuse the technology.

Banting himself may have been inspired by tales of nineteenth-century fur trappers in North America confronted with a low-carb regime, though not exactly by choice. They called it "rabbit starvation." Without carbs or fat, subsisting on ultra-lean wild meat in freezing northern climates where vegetation was scarce, trappers could eat even a whole deer and still essentially starve to death, as their bodies broke down tissue in desperation to fuel themselves. The all-the-lean-meat-you-can-eat diet killed off many backwoods entrepreneurs, though not those who understood the proper countermeasures (learned from Native Americans)—a slab of fat-rich beaver tail and some available vegetable matter, like tender inner spruce bark stripped off the tree and boiled up almost like pasta.

BUONO CARBS

Grains have been a worldwide staple for ten millennia, and it's no wonder when you consider all the health benefits of carbohydrates (and the dangerous effects of going without them). The *good* carbs are complex, nutrient-dense, fiber rich and slower to break down in the body, releasing their energy at more consistent rates. Full of vitamins, minerals, micronutrients and antioxidants, "goodfellas" like whole grains, vegetables, beans, legumes and fruit are the healthiest food choices you can make. Besides being ideally nourishing, they are also delicious.

Various studies have linked eating plenty of the right carbs with a decreased risk of heart disease, stroke, diabetes, certain digestive disorders and some types of cancer. The B vitamins whole grains provide are important for skin, hair, eye and liver health. They also help maintain normal digestive processes, as does the fiber found in complex carbs, which protects digestive health, including helping to prevent colon cancer. Some of the phytochemicals found in whole grains have been found to slow or stop the growth of cancer cells. A four-year study conducted at Tufts University demonstrated that carb-rich foods high in potassium and magnesium, such as oats, brown rice and spinach, balance blood acidity and increase bone density.

Despite all this good news about carbs, the average American doesn't even get one serving a day of whole grains (despite government recommendations for three or more daily), while as many as one in three say they are avoiding carbs. (For better or worse, most people who cut refined carbs fail to do so significantly, still eating up to six times as many as recommended by low-carb diets.) Studies show American adults average only half the official recommendation of fiber for good health and disease prevention (25–38 grams per day). People are growing fat on plenty of bad carbs rather than getting slim on the good carbs their bodies need. *Che peccato*—what a shame!

The biggest secret about carbs amidst all the low-carb weight loss hype is that eating the right carbs will help you *control* your weight!

RICH AND WHITE

Plato advocated whole meal bread made from locally grown wheat as a key to living healthfully into old age as far back as 400 BCE, but the Egyptian philosopher Athenaeus (c. 200 CE) documented that the preferred bread of the wealthy was white. Sifting ground wheat by hand through silk filters was a painstaking procedure that ensured precious white flour and white bread were reserved as luxuries of the upper crust.

White bread remained a status symbol for centuries, even after the Industrial Revolution made refined white flour more readily available than swarthy peasant whole meal. Scientists in the 1920s finally identified the nutritional benefits of whole grain flour after rampant outbreaks of beriberi, pellagra and other vitamin deficiency diseases plagued the United States as a result of diets heavy with white flour and bread. Yet white bread never lost the luster it gained from its early association with royalty and the exclusive dinner tables of the wealthy.

Being fat has also long been associated with being rich, and it's no coincidence that, historically, it was rich people who were eating all those refined carbs!

Recent medical studies show carbohydrates to be very valuable as metabolic aids in reducing weight: The body burns seven times more calories when converting complex carbs into body fat than it does when converting dietary fat into body fat. And scientists know that the more whole grains you eat, the lower and slower your weight gain over the years will be. A study at the Harvard School of Public Health followed 27,000 people between ages 40 and 75 for eight years and concluded that "middle-age spread" was curtailed by more than a pound for every 40 grams of whole grains eaten each day—about the amount in a Diet Code serving of bread or pasta.

The fiber content of carb-based foods is a major reason they are good for weight control. All high-fiber foods, including fruits and vegetables, will help you to lose weight and then maintain a healthy weight. First of all, fiber itself effectively has no calories, since the body doesn't absorb it. Beyond that, foods with fiber in them make you feel full and keep you feeling full for longer, so you eat less, and less often, for the simple reason that you aren't hungry for more. Foods with fiber in them take longer to eat, since they usually require more chewing. So eating them buys you some time to recognize when you have had enough. They also take longer to digest, which is why the satisfaction of eating them sticks with you until your next meal. Eat "broken" carbs, however, and you just want to keep on eating.

Besides the help you get from fiber, B vitamins, which abound in whole grains, also help regulate your appetite. Complex carbs actually add most of the flavor, texture, variety and color to your meals. After a properly balanced meal including the once-dreaded carbs, you feel satisfied aesthetically, physiologically and sensually. You won't already be looking for the next morsel the way you are when you are dining on industricarbs that turn straight to sugar in your body.

We all know dietary deprivation will guarantee the ultimate failure of any way of eating for the simple reason that you won't stick with your plan. By including carbs in your diet as this book describes, you'll avoid that trap.

MAKING CARBS WORK FOR YOU: THE GLYCEMIC INDEX, NET CARBS AND GLYCEMIC LOAD

You do need to be smart about carbs; even a baker can't in good conscience tell you to go crazy with the white bread (though the Italian ones may be able to impart some classic Old Country cooking tricks that can make healthy carbs even easier on your blood sugar. See chapter 6 for details).

To make that workable, look at the interaction between the glycemic index and the net carb index, which both quantify the effects of various carbs on your body, and the limitations and flaws in those systems.

The glycemic index (GI), developed at the University of Toronto in 1990, has been the "tommy gun" of the low-carb crowd ever since. Basically, it ranks foods according to how quickly they are converted into glucose (blood sugar) during digestion. Carb-free fats rate a zero (0), while glucose itself is a perfect 100. Proteins can break down to form glucose, but the process is long and irregular, ranking them extremely low. Therefore, all carbs appear "worse" than fat or proteins. Low-GI foods are less processed and higher in fiber and include fresh fruits, beans, whole grains and partial protein carbs, such as dairy products. Foods with high-GI ratings—mostly refined foods devoid of the fiber in complex carbs—elevate blood sugar levels and raise your risk for type 2 diabetes. Low-GI foods like yogurt, plums and lentils presumably cause less metabolic riot than high-GI foods like sugar syrups, instant rice and jelly beans.

That's all well and good until certain oddities appear. Potatoes (94) rank worse than potato chips (54). Carrots (92) look more dangerous than cola (63). Table sugar (68) comes out significantly lower than corn flakes (92). A real head-scratcher is a Snickers bar, which at 44 beats out brown rice (50) and raw oat bran (59)!

The GI can easily be manipulated to make even natural carbs look bad, but it's that peanut-packed candy bar that holds the key to a significant loophole within the index. Peanuts rank very low (13), and the cocoa and fat in the chocolate even lower (0), offsetting the sugary caramel. The pairing of fat and protein with carbs—or low-GI carb foods with high-GI carb foods—keeps the total GI from soaring. This is the science behind Diet Code Principle #2 ("Just Two It"—see chapter 6) and key components of both the Apprentice and Journeyman strategies (explained in detail in chapter 7).

You can do the same yourself with any good carb. A slice of bread spread with farm butter or peanut butter or topped with a hunk of cheese moderates the effect of the carbs on blood sugar.

Traditional cuisines all feature such pairings, such as cereal and milk, rice and fish, and bread and olive oil, which thereby tap into proper metabolic pathways. These are known as *companatico—* companions—in Italy, especially in reference to what goes with bread.

Still, the GI concept can reinforce smart food choices when you are working on your weight. A review of 16 studies on the GI showed that people ate less when they ate low-GI whole grains, fruits and vegetables as compared to eating high-GI boxed and bagged refined carbs. The low-GI foods left people feeling more satisfied and less hungry.

Low-GI foods are a natural fit for your body. Food is meant to take its time going through your long digestive tract; the tract is long to give food time to break down completely. Low-GI foods move more slowly through the system, taking longer to digest and reaching further into the small intestine, where cells that trigger your body's own appetite suppressants live.

The GI, however, was never meant to be the last word on choosing carbohydrates. For one thing, it's an oversimplification. It considers in isolation something that never happens in isolation in real life. Foods consumed together interact in the digestive system. How much you eat of any given food also affects its impact on your body. Ideally, you'd want to know the complete impact on the body of the total meal.

Putting food fiber into the equation restores some sense of proportion. Dr. Atkins promoted this as "net carbs," which calculates how many carbs, unbound by fiber, are in the food by subtracting grams of fiber (which the body doesn't absorb) from the number of total carbs. This reflects the reality that the body does not handle all carbs the same way. Whole foods have lower net carbs, which is why foods like pears and whole grain bread maintain their good standing in the nutrition pantheon; they have net carb counts that offset their GIs.

By now, the idea of net carbs has been thoroughly exploited in the creation of "FrankenFoods" full of chemical substitutes for carbs. The body doesn't take in these fake carbs the same way it doesn't take in fiber, but the similarities end there. So I'm all for personal net carb counting as a gauge of smart carb choices, but don't let the chemists do it for you.

Glycemic load (GL) is a more accurate representation of how food effects human biology. You get it by multiplying the glycemic index by net carbs. This addresses the discrepancies in GI ratings raised earlier by taking into account the quantity of food involved and the interworking of foods eaten together. GL tells you how what you eat acts on the body.

The "Revised International Table of Glycemic Index (GI) and Glycemic Load (GL) Values—2002" gives a fuller perspective than considering GI alone. On it you can learn that a serving of carrots has about a third the GL of soda. Whole meal bread has half the load of white bread, and muesli-type cereals have half that of commercial cereal flakes. Full-fat yogurt is easier on the system than reduced-fat varieties, and whole fruit rates better for you than extracted juices.

And Leonardo's beans? They are one of the most effective foods you can eat. A half-pound serving has a low GL (approximately 11), five times less than that Snickers bar by weight.

Indigenous cultures worldwide developed preparations and combinations of carb-rich foods that meet modern lab standards for healthy GL. From obscure African *ga kenkey* (fermented cornmeal), Australian Aboriginal desert oak seed bread, Indian *dokla* (fermented steamed wheat and chickpea cake) or Pima mesquite cake to the more familiar Lebanese hummus or Latin American corn tortilla with pinto beans and tomato salsa, traditional ethnic cuisines evolved food smarts.

Sharing the old ways and the old foods offers the means to fix a fractured planet more than reliance on fads, clinical trials and political power plays does.

EAT FAT, STAY THIN

One of the great lines in *The Godfather* belongs to Clemenza; after a roadside hit, he tells his associate, "Leave the gun; take the cannoli." I'm no wiseguy, but on this point, I'm with him. I eat several of those Sicilian pastries a week, and they don't budge my weight. In fact, I'm sure they help me stay where I want to be on the scale.

I make my cannoli the way they deserve to be made, with full-fat ricotta and mascarpone. Those Italian cheeses are specifically high in calcium, a mineral proven to accelerate weight loss. Besides, my cannoli have gotten rave reviews from none other than Frank Serpico (the erstwhile NYC undercover cop who famously stood alone against corruption in the department during the *Goodfellas* era). By the way, Mr. Serpico is an eloquent and *lean* advocate of cannoli. Few of us are ever going to have Frank's "stugots," but in my own small way I'm trying to be a stand-up guy, too, making authentic cannoli, saying no to both fat and carb repression. Leave the fat-free frozen yogurt; take the cannoli.

Having fat in your diet is no more a cause for excess weight than having carbs is—again, as long as you get the right kind. The right kinds of natural fats also don't cause heart disease or cancer (though the wrong kinds—artificially altered—can). Fat, in fact, keeps your heart working well and your cholesterol levels healthy. Good fats raise your levels of good cholesterol (high-density lipoproteins, or HDL) *and* lower the bad (low-density lipoproteins, or LDL) and total cholesterol levels. Good fats decrease your triglyceride levels. They fight inflammation in the arteries, keeping them flexible and reducing blood clots. That is, eating natural fats *decreases* your risk of heart disease.

What's really dangerous about fat in your diet is not having enough. Fat-free meat, dairy or carbs (whose good oils are removed with the germ during refining) are all destructive to our organs and physiology, essentially starving us. A host of functions shut down, such as the ability to absorb many vitamins and minerals, but bluntly, we simply dry out. Imagine driving a car with no oil for the engine or grease for the chassis: The vehicle literally grinds down and seizes up. Nonfat dairy products, stripped of their natural fats and homogenized, thereby destroying the natural size of their component particles, have similarly been shown to increase the scarring of blood vessels, leading to strokes, blindness, heart attacks and arthritis. Besides protecting your heart, your body also uses fat to build muscle, maintain cell membranes, manufacture hormones, grow skin, hair and nails and keep eyes healthy. Fats are crucial to brain structure and function, and whole fats keep you thinking clearly and can even fight depression.

Some fats even help you *burn* fat. The body uses good fats for energy (and tends to store bad fats as fat). A study published in the *International Journal of Obesity* in 2002 showed that the human body burns more fat during the five hours after a meal high in monounsaturated fats (as found in olives, avocados, nuts and seeds) than after a meal full of saturated fat. This was especially true in people who were overweight. A study done in 1997 showed that people taking 6 grams per day of fish oil supplement (a source of omega-3 essential fatty acids, which are also found in nuts and seeds) burned more fat for energy and stored more glucose in the muscles. Eating fat is actually one of your major weapons in the battle against the bulge.

In addition, fat has an effect on satiety—a long-lasting sensation of being full and satisfied. Besides which, fats make food taste good. Low-fat regimens always leave you feeling hungry and unsatisfied. Even worse, people on low-fat diets tend to replace the fat with bad carbs, a double whammy for the body.

THE BEST FATS

The fats with the greatest health benefits are the omega-3 fatty acids and monounsaturated fats. You should get them the same way Leonardo would have: in olives and olive oil; almonds and other nuts; dark, leafy greens and (if he didn't forswear flesh) fish (especially eel, which was popular and relatively easy to get inland in the fifteenth century).

There is another group of essential fatty acids (deemed "essential" because the body can't manufacture them and must take them in via the diet), omega-6s, but since these are found in the vegetable oils used pervasively in food processing in this country (including canola, corn, safflower, soybean and sunflower oils), Americans get more than enough. We get so much, in fact, that we upset the ideal balance between omega-6s and omega-3s in our bodies, getting 20 times as much of the former as the latter, when the ideal ratio is no greater than 2:1. And 2:1 is what has been throughout most of history, until the relatively recent advent of pervasive processed food, seemingly all of which is dunked in omega-6 oils. Our bodies are forced to operate

---

GET YOUR OMEGA-3S HERE

It used to be that meat from grass-fed and wild animals was a good source of omega-3s, but that's no longer true of meat from today's pellet-fed animals. You can rely on these foods instead.

Cold-Water Fish
- salmon
- lake trout
- herring
- sardines
- tuna
- anchovies
- mackerel
- bluefish
- turbot

Nuts and Seeds (And Their Oils)
- walnuts
- flaxseed
- hemp seed
- pumpkin seed

And . . .
- omega-3–enriched eggs
- dark, leafy greens (at 1 gram per 6-ounce serving, this won't compare to fish or nuts, but it's still a significant source and the best you'll find among vegetables)

far from optimally as they use these fatty acids acquired in such lop-sided proportion to create the full range of fats they need to support healthy cells and tissues. You don't want to get rid of omega-6s alto-gether—they have excellent anti-inflammatory properties—but at the same time, you blunt their effectiveness by overdosing yourself. As always, what's optimal involves balance and proportion.

SAT FATS

In most of the diet books that have proliferated over the last decades, this would be the "shakedown" section highlighting the worst of all the forbidden demons. But saturated fat, and the animal foods and occasional plant foods (coconut and palm oils) it is found in, have got-ten a bad rap. You don't officially need to eat it, since the body can manufacture saturated fat out of carbohydrates, but it is the only fat that protects the heart and is necessary for many structures in your cells. Stearic acid, for example, a saturated fat found in beef and chocolate, makes a beeline for cell membranes, where it is used to repair and maintain them. Caprylic acid combats the growth of unwanted yeast, and lauric acid has antiviral and antibacterial proper-ties. Saturated fat from farm butter, eggs and grass-fed beef actually increases good cholesterol, lowers triglycerides and aids calcium absorption and omega-3 fatty acid utilization.

BAD FATS

Now we come to the real *malandrino* (bad guy): trans fat. Trans fat is what you get from hydrogenated or partially hydrogenated oils—liquid oils with hydrogen forced into them to make them solid at room temperature, such as margarine and shortening, and stable in packaged foods. With the fat thus artificially transformed from its natural state into a laboratory creation, it not only keeps products "fresh" on the shelf indefinitely (do you really want to eat something that never spoils?) but also increases your risk of obesity, clogged arteries, heart disease, diabetes, stroke, cancer, immune system dysfunction and birth defects. Trans fat increases total and LDL (bad) cholesterol and decreases HDL (good) cholesterol. In short, trans fats do what saturated fats have for too long been accused of doing.

Cut the commercial processed foods out of your life—cookies, crackers, chips, cakes, pies, shortening, breads, margarine—and you'll be rid of 75% of the trans fat in the average American's diet as well as the worst carbohydrate forms you can eat. (Baked goods handcrafted by artisans are a different story altogether.)

ONE RECIPE YOU *DON'T* WANT

Refined carbs or fats are unhealthy, especially when eaten exclusively or to excess, *and so are all the other refined or fragmented food forms*. At this point, the American food supply is so altered by industrial demands and chemical additives that the very system we should be relying on to nourish us directly contributes to poor nutrition and weight gain. What's easiest to come by are nutritionally deficient foods. We eat (and drink) more and more foods with less and less nutritional benefits. We move less. We live the "more is better" American dream when it comes to what we mindlessly put on our plates and into our mouths. Carbs or no carbs, fats or no fats, that is a recipe for disaster.

CHAPTER FIVE

Fundamental Foods and Functional Nutrition

Study mathematics, and do not build without foundations.
—LEONARDO DA VINCI

*A land of wheat, and barley, and vines, and fig trees, and
pomegranates; a land of oil olive, and honey; A land wherein
thou shalt eat bread without scarceness.*
—DEUTERONOMY (THE FIFTH BOOK OF MOSES) 8:8–9
(DESCRIBING THE PROMISED LAND)

Humans evolved eating the most nutrient-dense foods available. A diet of these foods charges the metabolism. Yet in our contemporary consumer culture, with thousands of selections at hand, the bulk of our modern diet is calorie-dense but nutrient-sparse. Two of the three most popular "vegetables" in America are French fries and iceberg lettuce, both of which have virtually no nutritional value. (We'll soon get to the third, tomato sauce, which is actually among the best things you can eat.)

The Diet Code, on the other hand, is based on the most potent foods on the planet, as readily available now as in Leonardo's fifteenth century. I call these Fundamental Foods, and they should be the core of your diet. They provide the richest tastes, the most nutrients per ounce and the greatest benefit to your metabolism. They are the best foods for reaching and maintaining a healthful weight and the best choice for overall good health.

The Diet Code focuses on the Fundamental Foods in the service of functional nutrition—that is, choosing not just good food but optimal nutrient sources. The idea is to get the most out of every bite. Nutrient-dense foods satisfy the body on a deep level. This automatically leads to eating smaller portions and, in turn, to natural weight loss.

Choosing the right food (Fundamental Foods) is the first of two core ideas that make The Diet Code work. The second, combining these foods in the right proportions, will be explained in more detail in chapter 7.

FUNDAMENTAL FOODS

The list of Fundamental Foods that follows is short—only six basic vegetables, for instance. After introducing the Fundamental Foods in the following two lists, I'll give you a bit more detail about each food group. These lists are not meant to exclude the many other natural, nutritious foods available but rather to spotlight the common ones you should not do without. The Diet Code promotes the Fundamental Vegetables, for instance, for their overall nutrient density, but by no means should you ignore the great range of other vegetables, including string beans and snow peas, summer squash, celery, fennel, artichokes, cucumbers, mushrooms, radishes and eggplant. Choose *most* of your foods from these lists, however, and you'll be well on your way to living The Diet Code.

Leafy Greens

This is the single most important group of vegetables, yet it is also the one most commonly missing from the average diet. Greens are one food I cannot live without, and would not want to. If you're one of the people who has not yet discovered the many wonders of these vegetables, the time is now! It may require a bit of new knowledge to prepare them in such a way that you will truly enjoy them, but once you learn, you'll never go back. I used to tend raised garden beds

FUNDAMENTAL CARBOHYDRATES

Choose from these most nutritionally dense and metabolically powerful carbs each day.

Vegetables
- **leafy greens:** cabbage, kale, broccolini, raab, escarole, chard, spinach, choi, sea vegetables, kimchi, sauerkraut
- **onions:** leeks, scallions, garlic
- **legumes:** lentils, chickpeas, beans, peas, miso, tempeh (fermented soy)
- **Italian salad greens:** parsley, dandelion, arugula, cress, endive, valeriana
- **asparagus**
- **peppers**
- **tomato sauce**
- **orange vegetables:** acorn, butternut and buttercup winter squashes, pumpkin, carrots, beets, sweet potatoes

Grains
- **breads:** handcrafted whole meal sourdough
- **whole grains:** bulgur, farro, quinoa, spelt, brown rice, barley, millet, oats, corn, rye
- **pasta:** artisanal durum, spelt, buckwheat, kamut and quinoa varieties

Other
- *dolce:* seasonal fresh fruits (especially berries), figs, prunes, dried apricots, raisins, raw honey, dark chocolate, beer, wine

holding about 30 varieties of greens, including four types of kale—some growing 3 feet high. One of my favorites was the wild and weedy stinging nettle. Nettles' flavor is reminiscent of oysters, which made them a prime candidate for inclusion in a potato leek soup cooked with a bit of smoked bacon or pancetta.

FUNDAMENTAL PROTEINS AND FATS

Most protein-rich foods also contain fat, and many foods with good fats also contain protein. Therefore, I've included both on this selected list of Fundamental Foods that should round out your meals.

Animal Sources
- **fish:** especially cold-water, fatty ocean varieties, like anchovy, sardine, smelt, herring, mackerel, salmon, halibut, tuna
- **poultry and meat:** grass-fed natural (free-range and organic, especially antibiotic free) chicken, turkey, lamb and beef
- **dairy:** lacto-fermented products (yogurt, kefir, cottage cheese, ricotta, crème fraiche), artisanal cheeses, butter

Plant Sources
- avocados, olives, olive oil, grapeseed oil
- **nuts and seeds:** almonds, walnuts, hemp, flaxseed, sesame, sunflower, pumpkin seeds and their oils

Greens come in four major types, representing the cole, beet, mustard and lettuce families:

- The *cole* crops include cabbage, kale, collards and Brussels sprouts. Additionally, broccoli and cauliflower are flower heads bred (by Italian horticulturalists) from this family. Broccolini is a smaller, more tender and peppery version of broccoli with an older lineage, and I find it a much superior vegetable.
- The *beet* family includes Swiss chard, spinach, oriental choi varieties and, of course, tasty beet greens themselves.

Vegetables from the above two families are the ones most often pickled or fermented to form sauerkraut (which the Romans barreled and ate 2,000 years ago) and Korean kimchi.

- The *mustard* family includes raab and mustard greens in both European and Asian varieties.
- From the *lettuce* family I choose sturdy types, like radicchio, endive and the more familiar romaine (which are fabulous grilled), as well as escarole, a traditional Italian soup green (often accompanied by a poached egg and corn bread).

Italian salad greens, such as parsley, young dandelion, arugula, cress, frisée and valeriana (a mild buttery leaf also known as corn salad, lamb's lettuce or mache), pack more nutritional punch than conventional lettuce and make cleansingly bitter or pungent seasonal splashes at your dinner table.

SALAD: THE UNNECESSARY "HEALTH FOOD"

The ritual "vegetable," even for many nutritionally savvy Americans, is the side salad. We keep ordering the typical iceberg lettuce/mealy tomato abomination available everywhere from burger joints and taco houses to Asian restaurants (where a cup of green tea would easily give you more benefits than an American side salad). We've mistakenly deified this pointless bowl, making the salad bar a shrine of health, nutritionally deceptive and compromised though it is with calorie-laden gelatins, fake bacon and creamy dressings.

Now, there's nothing wrong with a good salad, but we've diverged from the *sallet* days of our Masonic founders Washington, Franklin and Jefferson and the earlier Roman *salata*—dishes that got their names from the Latin noun for salt. Old-time salads

(continued on next page)

were salted field herbs: shoots, stems, leaves, flower heads, blossoms and tendrils, both raw and cooked (see chapter 10 for some recipes along these lines).

At Sophia's, first-time customers as conditioned to the ubiquitous salad as anyone else often ask, somewhat puzzled, "Don't you have any greens?" When I point out braised chard with leeks, rice-and-lemon-stuffed vine leaves or sliver-sliced cabbage and parsley salad with anise and caper dressing, I often get blank stares. Enthusiasm starts after one taste and then continues as patrons return time and again for the real flavor and bodily "lift" they claim to get after eating a side of chard or Italian slaw.

All greens are not created equal. Consider the spectrum, ranging from iceberg through romaine to kale. (The comparison below is based on analyses from the *Nutrition Almanac,* fifth edition, by Lavon Dunne.) In equal-size servings,

- romaine has about twice the protein of iceberg, and kale has almost four times as much.
- romaine has over seven times as much vitamin A as iceberg, and kale has almost twenty-four times as much.
- romaine has twice iceberg's niacin and calcium, and kale has over five times as much.
- romaine has four times the vitamin C of iceberg, and kale has eighteen times as much.
- additionally, kale has well over twice the level of potassium found in the lettuces. Kale has over three times the calories of lettuce––a good thing in vegetables, because it makes you feel full. If you're mindlessly eating lettuce as filler, at least choose the more robust romaine. Make the switch altogether to dark leafy greens, and you will feel the energy boost that mindful, and functional, nutrition can make.

Onions

The allium family is one of the oldest staple foods of humans. Winter storing onions are cured within their papery husks, but many varieties are eaten for both bulb and stem, like scallions and the ancient, high-calcium leek of which the Romans were so fond. Onions (and garlic) may be considered the second most important vegetable after greens for their versatility and overall nutritional contributions of vitamin A, B_6, phosphorus, potassium, zinc and protein.

Legumes

Beans have protein, fiber and iron, making them good for building muscle, stoking metabolism and feeling full after you eat—in short, good for losing weight. An 8-ounce, or 1-cup, serving averages a substantial 15 grams of protein, and about twice that amount of carbs—a nearly perfect Diet Code ratio. Beans have almost no fat, which is why so many traditional dishes across all cultures add cheese, sour cream, avocado or bacon to bean dishes.

Lentils, ceci (chickpeas), black-eyed peas and fava were the original beans of the Mediterranean, while runner and shell beans, like lima, flageolet, white kidney (cannellini), red and black, pinto and borlotti were adopted from the Americas.

Soybeans are another ancient food—this time from Asia—of the utmost importance for the "second brain," fostering digestive order, healthy blood and muscle power. Soybeans are a complete protein, providing all required amino acids, but have no cholesterol or saturated fat. Optimal nutrition comes from the two traditional fermented preparations, miso and tempeh. (See the fermented foods box on p. 89.) Miso is a bean paste used in soups and sauce bases that makes an instant broth I start every day with, but also is a perfect quick preface to any meal (see recipe on p. 267). Tempeh is a sprouted bean cake that packs a load of protein (18 grams per 4-ounce serving). My favorite preparation is a grilled tempeh burger (see recipe on p. 294) that can make a hot sandwich or substitute for a cut of steak.

Asparagus

In a class by itself, this nutrient-packed vegetable is high in protein, vitamins and minerals—particularly iron, potassium, magnesium and zinc. It's been grown commercially for hundreds of years in Italy and is harvested as a shoot. I have fond memories of my grandfather patiently spading a new bed for asparagus (3 feet deep!) and "seasoning" it with hoof, horn or bone meal. He never harvested a planting before the third year; this patience paid off in thick and tender spears.

GET MY VITAMINS?

Under ideal conditions, vitamin supplementation would be unnecessary. Eating The Diet Code variety of foods, selected for maximum nutrition, should provide the body with all the nutrients it needs. But in today's world, stress, skipped meals and denatured food quality undermine the ideal. Foods, organic or not, are nutritionally depleted thanks to poor soil, processing and delays from harvest to table. Besides, if you've been eating anything that even somewhat resembles the typical American diet, your body hasn't been properly nourished for a long time, and you're going to have some catching up to do.

You can provide yourself a bit of insurance by taking a high-quality multivitamin that hasn't been chemically produced. Avoid cheap, synthetic drugstore vitamins, choosing instead "food sourced" or "nature sourced" multis from a health food store.

These are natural compressed or extracted food elements rather than chemical versions.

Lab-made supplements may have inappropriate dosages or combinations of nutrients, may be rendered ineffective by processing or may be made from materials your body can't really absorb. Chemical vitamins may be enantiomeric, or mirror-image compounds. Picture the body's receptor sites for nutrients as the right hand on which only the "right glove" compound will fit properly. A cheaply produced "left glove" version can be sold under the same name as the nutrient you desire, but it's unable to fit and function authentically in your body.

Natural vitamins may be harder to find and seem more expensive when compared with synthetics, but in the long run, they are actually more economical because they can and will be absorbed and used by your body. Besides, after a year or so on The Diet Code, you'll only need a fraction of the recommended doses anyway, since the supplement will be simply a backup plan to a diet naturally rich in everything your body needs to function at peak capacity, both physically and mentally. At that point, stick with the quality vitamins but halve the dosage, or take them every other day rather than daily.

Peppers

Potent sources of vitamins A and C, peppers were an important food in the Americas 500 years ago, even though they were merely potted ornamentals in Italy for another two centuries. Although Leonardo would not have known them (or tomatoes, potatoes, coffee or cocoa) as food, since their introduction they have evolved as a mainstay of Mediterranean cuisine.

Tomatoes

This is one of only two fruits or vegetables whose nutritional value *increases* with processing (the other being corn). Tomato paste is arguably the most nutrient-dense fruit on the planet. It has the same amount of protein by weight as the mighty asparagus (over 4 grams per 5 ounces) and about half the valuable glutamic acid of beef. Tomatoes are a key source of lycopene, an antioxidant that protects against heart disease and cancer. Concentrated in sauce and paste, tomatoes contain whopping amounts of vitamins A, B, C, E, niacin, folic and pantothenic acids, calcium, iron, magnesium, manganese, phosphorus, potassium, selenium and zinc. The garden-ripe fresh fruit is divine, but to really stoke your weight loss, stock the sauce.

Orange Vegetables

These meaty, carb-rich roots, tubers and gourds are bursting with vitamin A and are robust sources of potassium, phosphorus and calcium. One cup of winter squash, pumpkin or sweet potato has about half the carbs as does an equivalent serving of pasta, bulgur or rice, so consider substituting these sustaining veggies for grains at a meal.

Dolce

Sweets in Leonardo's time primarily meant fresh fruit. Honey, dried fruit and preserves were secondary, and sugar was a rare condiment, much like pepper or other imported spices. Returning to such a pattern would be a significant move toward optimal health and weight, though it is bound to be shocking to modern taste buds that are so bombarded with sweetness.

If you scale back on the added sugars in your overall diet, you will soon rediscover the inherent sweetness in carb-rich foods—fruits, of course, but also vegetables, whole grains and even plain yogurt! And once you are at that place, the occasional use of any added (natural) sweetener will not negatively affect your health or weight.

When it comes to choosing dolce, your best bet by far is the same as Leonardo's default option: fresh fruit. The word *fruit* comes from

IN DEFENSE OF CANE SUGAR

For baking, I often use cane sugar. It adds structural value, like loft in cakes and crispness in cookies. The texture of things made with sugar is irreproducible, and the taste of sugar is really clean—it lets other flavors come through without interference.

That's the technical viewpoint of a baker. But I do the same thing at home as I do in my shop, and I expect you will want to as well. Cane sugar, demon of upstanding nutritionists everywhere, has a certain place in my kitchen. What it does, it does well, and it just can't be replaced by anything else.

I choose less refined versions—turbinado or demerara—keeping in line with The Diet Code line of "the less refined, the better." And while I'm not a fanatic about avoiding cane sugar, I use it sparingly. I guess I'm pulling down the average of the typical American, who consumes more sugar in one year than Leonardo did in the nearly seven decades of his life. (And that's only counting the sugar that's in soft drinks and juices!)

What I *am* fanatic about is eliminating high-fructose corn syrup, which more and more frequently is used in place of cane sugar in commercially prepared foods, especially the vast majority of soft drinks and juices. About two-thirds of the high-fructose corn syrup ingested in the United States today comes from beverages like those. And that's two-thirds of a staggering amount: Consumption of high-fructose corn syrup in this country increased 1,000% between 1970 and 1990, according to a study published in the *American Journal of Clinical Nutrition* in 2004.

(continued on next page)

It's no coincidence that the rate of obesity has doubled since 1970, too, now that fully 10% of our total caloric intake is from high-fructose corn syrup. This particular sugar substitute, besides being ultra-refined, is addictive and especially fattening. This syrup is handled through an entirely different metabolic pathway in the human body than is sugar. Sugar is metabolized as grains, fruit and vegetables are. But high-fructose corn syrup has a different chemical configuration that the body doesn't recognize as a legitimate sugar. Because of that, it's not used directly for energy but is shunted to the liver and converted into fat. And because the body hasn't registered having received sugar as fuel, we don't feel satisfied, so we increase our consumption. Furthermore, it does not, like natural sugars, spur the production of leptin, which regulates appetite, so again, we consume more.

the Latin *fruor,* "I delight in," and so you should! For peak enjoyment, choose among seasonal melons, plums, pears, peaches, nectarines, bananas (the most commonly eaten fruit in the United States, with apples close behind), apples, citrus, pineapples, mangoes, grapes and cherries. Berries of all varieties are generally recognized as being the most nutrient-dense and are particularly packed with beneficial antioxidants.

Dried fruit is a concentrated source of sweetness. Eat only a quarter of what you would eat of the same fresh fruit—1.5 ounces, or a quarter of a cup dry, for example, versus 6 ounces (about 1 cup) fresh. On the flip side, because it is such a concentrated source of sweetness yet still a whole food full of nutrients and fiber, dried fruit makes a good choice for sweetening recipes. Similarly, unsweetened whole fruit syrups, juices and concentrates, like apple butter, are also better sweetening agents than grain syrups made from rice or barley, as they have lower glycemic indexes.

Raw honey may be the oldest natural concentrated sweetener and is still the most nutritious, particularly when it comes to minerals. Another best choice is agave cactus nectar, a premium sweetener that tastes like a fine-grade maple syrup, has a very low GI (11) and can replace honey or sugar using just three-quarters of the amount. Other natural sugars, like real maple syrup, molasses and evaporated cane juice (natural brown sugar) or cane sugar can also be used judiciously. As always, organic is the best bet, no matter what the particular sweetener.

Chocolate

One of the most nutritious dolce you can choose is chocolate. Its antioxidant polyphenols, particularly flavonoids, help prevent diabetes, heart disease and some kinds of cancer. Studies (done in Italy, naturally!) show that eating dark chocolate daily can lower blood pressure and improve the body's ability to metabolize sugar. Other studies demonstrate that dark chocolate reduces blood clots and clumps, much the way aspirin does, and that dark chocolate increases good cholesterol levels and stops bad cholesterol from wreaking havoc in its usual way (by oxidizing).

It's cacao beans we have to thank for the flavonoid supply; a Cornell study showed cocoa has more antioxidants than two other famously excellent sources: red wine and green tea. Other green and red fruits and vegetables also contain flavonoids, and chocolate shouldn't be your only source of them, but you're unlikely to find another source as luxurious!

You can't count all chocolate as health food, however. The darker the chocolate, generally speaking, the higher the nutrient level. White chocolate, for example, is devoid of flavonoids (and study volunteers given white rather than dark chocolate showed no change in blood pressure or diabetes risk for this reason). Processing can reduce the amount of flavonoids; some is lost while fermenting cocoa beans and some when alkali is used in making the chocolate (a fact that may or may not be noted on the label). The higher the cocoa content, the better. The percentage of cocoa is now often proudly proclaimed on the labels of better chocolates; look for at least 60 to 70%. Organically grown, minimally processed dark chocolate is your best bet.

An appropriate serving size of chocolate is just 0.5 to 1 ounce, but if you choose high quality and savor each bite, even that small amount should be as satisfying as it is nutritious. The Diet Code easily accommodates chocolate, even daily chocolate; plan ahead for dessert, count it into your carbohydrate portion and balance it with other macronutrients appropriately (as described in chapter 10). Leonardo may have had to do without chocolate, since it wasn't introduced from the New World until the middle of the 1500s, but there's no reason you have to!

Red Wine

In Renaissance times, sugars comprised a much less significant proportion of overall carbohydrates in the diet than they do today. But of the sugars people did get, a good portion came from wine. It's probably not a bad pattern to imitate, at least for those of us who enjoy a glass with dinner. That fits right into The Diet Code plan, and in addition to being compatible with weight loss, studies from around the world show that in moderation, wine can help reduce the risk of heart disease, type 2 diabetes, osteoporosis, dementia and stroke. That's thanks in large part to the antioxidant flavonoids it contains, alcohol's ability to keep arteries flexible and the presence of good cholesterol–raising polyphenols. Red wine has eight times as many flavonoids as does white wine (for nonwine drinkers, a similar level shows up in grape juice). It also improves digestion and has antibiotic properties.

The heart-protective effects of red wine usually get all the press, but I want to highlight the benefits of dry red wine (low in residual sugar) in diabetes in particular. The theory goes that alcohol improves glucose tolerance, moderating the effect of eating carbohydrates on blood sugar levels. In diabetics, the need for this may have reached a critical level, but the effect is beneficial for everyone and is key not only for good health and high energy levels but also for weight loss.

You're going to need to modify the quantity of wine in your diet from the Renaissance standard, however. If Leonardo was typical of his neighbors, wine was a basic daily beverage, and he probably drank almost a liter of it a day—some experts say up to a half gallon. It was often diluted with water, but still! The Diet Code calls for a 5-ounce serving, or just what you'd expect to get if you bought a glass in a bar or restaurant. I enjoy a glass of chilled white wine, depending on what I'm eating with it and the time of year (it's more of a warm-weather choice for me), but I usually drink red. I especially like dry red Tuscan wines like Chianti. In any case, I choose estate-made wines. As long as you avoid the generic, commercial, blended wines that don't really come from any one place in particular, there are many delicious but relatively inexpensive bottles to be had.

Beer

Red wine has gotten the most attention in the discussion of potential health benefits of alcohol and it is particularly high in antioxidants, but the truth is that alcohol in general, consumed in moderation, is good for most people. This finding was once so controversial that the medical community worked to suppress it, apparently fearing the public couldn't be trusted to tell the difference between having a drink and abusing alcohol (which entails a variety of disastrous health effects, of course). But by 1985, there was even a review article published in the journal *Drug and Alcohol Dependence* summarizing international data on the advantages of light to moderate alcohol intake. It primarily credits the way alcohol increases good cholesterol. Moderate alcohol consumption decreases the death rate from all causes, but especially heart-related ones. It also mentions, however, the silicon content in wine and beer, alcohol's blood-thinning properties, the relatively healthier diets that moderate drinkers tend to have and the stress reduction that comes from simply having a drink. Alcoholic beverages' antioxidant properties are also protective.

Many studies show, however, that like red wine, beer is more beneficial than other alcoholic beverages. In part, a similar explanation applies: Like red wine, beer contains antioxidant polyphenols, which are unrelated to alcohol content, that protect the heart. Besides cardiovascular benefits, beer has also been shown to help prevent (and slow) cancer, osteoporosis, diabetes and lifestyle-related diseases in general. Here again, the benefits don't come from the alcohol content. Beer provides a portion of the Recommended Daily Allowance of several vitamins and impressive amounts of important trace metals and minerals. When it comes to cancer prevention, research points to a variety of polyphenols derived from malt and hops, according to a review article by German scientists published in the *European Journal of Cancer* in 2005. A study published in the *Lancet* followed 111 healthy men in the Netherlands who had one glass of beer each day for three weeks. They experienced an increase in good cholesterol and a 30% increase in blood levels of vitamin B_6, which stimulates the immune system and protects blood vessels. Of particular interest to *The Diet Code* readers, a report from the Third International Conference on Food Factors in 2004 published in *Biofactors* heralded bitter substances derived from hops called isohumulones as helping prevent and reverse obesity as well as type 2 diabetes and improving cholesterol profiles and atherosclerosis.

In short, beer is good food. Dark beer is even better—it has three times the flavonoids of paler ale—so I most often choose Guinness, Murphy's or other stouts, especially in the winter. In doing so, I may be making the best choice of alcohol of all, at least for a man. A study published in 1997 in the *American Journal of Cardiology* of almost 4,000 patients belonging to a California HMO who were hospitalized for heart disease concluded that while beer, wine and liquor all provided heart-healthy benefits in moderation, beer showed the greatest benefits in men, while women benefited most from wine. Cheers!

Whole Grains

Grains run a close second to leafy greens in the list of most disregarded, untapped and nearly forgotten foodstuffs in America. Taking full advantage of this 10,000-year-old foundational food group as well as greens together would revolutionize the contemporary diet and reverse the ever-increasing trend toward obesity, not to mention our pill-popping dependence because of a huge variety of ills.

Quinoa, the ancient cereal of the Inca Empire, for example, is not only a good source of fiber but is also high in calcium and protein. And because it contains the amino acid lysine, which is usually low in grains, quinoa is a complete protein. It is also full of potassium, zinc, folic acid, iron, magnesium and B vitamins, particularly vitamin B_6. Quinoa is a leafy grain, so it is a good choice for those with food sensitivities, who often react to grassy grains, like corn and wheat. And it contains no gluten, so even people who cannot tolerate wheat, corn, rye, barley and oats can enjoy it.

Use a variety of grains in a range of preparations to take full advantage of their bounty. Make hot breakfast cereal (porridge) from cut (or Irish) oats, bulgur (toasted cracked wheat), millet or quinoa. Choose hulled barley, which is less refined and tastier than pearled, for soups. Boil up cornmeal into the very versatile Italian polenta. Brown rice and whole wheat couscous make great companions for grilled, roasted and braised meats and vegetables.

Rolled grain flakes of spelt, rye, barley and kamut also boil up, like oatmeal, into incredibly flavorful hot cereals and can even be combined into rich flourless muffins (see recipe on p. 269). And with old-fashioned rolled oats cooking in under two minutes, there is no excuse for avoiding a home-cooked breakfast or buying premade quick-cooking cereals.

Get at least one serving (¼ to ⅓ cup dry or ¾ to 1 cup cooked) daily of whole grains, and I mean *whole or cracked kernels*. Include them in one meal out of your five, for sure, and more if you can, alternating with pasta, bread and potatoes.

CERES

The Italians have literally worshipped grain from way back, personified in the form of Ceres, goddess of agriculture, fertility and grain. From her name we derive the word *cereal*. Ceres was the Roman goddess of soil, health and farming techniques, and, to be sure, the bread that was so often the end result of those efforts.

The annual Cerealia was held in her honor each April, celebrating the growth of crops and the prospect of a good harvest (Ceres willing). She was given her due in many ways throughout the year, whether the preharvest sacrifice of a fertile female pig or, as Cato suggested, a pumpkin. Either way, you'd want to offer her wine to go with that . . . the first fruits of any given yield were often dedicated to her as well. Images of Ceres often show her crowned with corn stalks, cradling sheaves of wheat. On one coin, she's shown wearing a modius, an instrument for measuring grain. Sometimes she herself appears to be growing out of the earth.

The Romans adopted Ceres in 496 BCE during a crisis—widespread famine—when it seemed only natural that they should appeal to a figure much like the Greek goddess Demeter in the interest of renewing their main source of food.

In our collective abandonment of grain foods, we've turned our backs on Ceres. In all other times and ages, malnutrition was mostly a function of famine or scarcity. Today, for the first time in human history, more people on the planet are overfed than underfed. Our overweight bodies bear witness to a new phenomenon, a *malnutrition of abundance*.

Pasta

As a baker, I like to claim a "Body by Bread." Sophia Loren, on the other hand, declared, "Everything you see I owe to pasta!" That's a lot of leverage for a lowly bowl of noodles.

Thirty million Italians can't be wrong: A poll (admittedly, one sponsored by the Union of Italian Pasta Producers) revealed that over half of Italians eat pasta *every day*—downing four times as much pasta per capita than Americans. It's worth noting, however, that Italians eat their pasta as one of several courses—meaning, in small portions at any given time—rather than as one big mountain of spaghetti, American style. The first appearance of pasta in Europe was probably the wide Latin noodle *laganum;* more refined forms don't seem to occur until about the ninth or tenth century CE in Italy. And for a thousand years, Italians have stayed slim, dining regularly on pasta—in Diet Code–sized portions (2 to 3 ounces dry, 6 to 8 ounces cooked).

Americans have misunderstood and misappropriated pasta just as they have all grain foods. Please, skip the cheap white pasta *and* the gritty, badly made whole wheat knock-offs. This is not the place for hard, modern whole wheat. Choose instead *artisanal* semolina (yellow

GUIDE TO MACRONUTRIENTS IN PASTAS

per 2-ounce (dry) serving (4–6 ounces or ¼–⅓ pound cooked)

Grain Type	Calories	Net Carbs (g)	Protein (g)	Fat (g)
Kamut	190	27	10	1.5
Spelt- and buckwheat-blend soba	200	35	9	1.5
Spelt	210	40	9	0.5
Kamut and quinoa blend	210	35	8	2
Quinoa	180	33	4	2
Durum semolina	200	38	7	0.5
Rice	200	44	3	0

PASTA NAMES

Italians have named pasta shapes for every facet of life, from the descriptive, practical and technical to the fanciful, farcical and beautiful. Here are some of my favorite examples, from the *Dictionary of Italian Food and Drink* by John Mariani.

Anchellini, "maidservants"
Barette, "little dribbles"
Cansonsei, "little britches"
Denti di caballo,
   "horse teeth"
Ditalini, "little toes"
Elice, "screws"
Farfalle, "butterflies"
Filini, "cat whiskers"
Gallanini, "floaters"
Gigantoni, "giants"
Gnudi, "nudes"
Gramigna, "grass"
Grandine, "hailstones"
Maltagliati, "badly cut"
Mandilli de saea, "silk
   handkerchiefs"
Maniche, "sleeves"

Marabini, "little rubies"
Matasse, "tangles"
Occhi di pernice,
   "partridge eyes"
Panzarotti, "little bellies"
Pappardelle, "gulp downs"
Ricci di donna,
   "lady's curls"
Strangolapreti,
   "priest stranglers"
Strichetti, "pinched"
Stringozzi, "big shoelaces"
Tagliatelle, "tresses"
Tempestini,
   "little snowfalls"
Umbilichi sacri,
   "sacred navels"

durum wheat) pasta, which is often shaped with old-style bronze dies. Also look for delicious blends of ancient whole grains, like quinoa, spelt, emmer and kamut, which make excellent, supple noodles (and, in the case of quinoa and spelt, provide complete protein). Another great choice is Ezekiel 4:9 brand complete protein sprouted multigrain pasta. Spelt and buckwheat noodles are also available in the Japanese forms, udon and soba.

Bread

Italians eat almost half a pound of bread per day in the service of maintaining their slim physiques. That's about 4.5 *billion* pounds of bread collectively consumed in Italy each year, according to Carol Field in *The Italian Baker*.

That's not just empty calories they are eating. Bread contains vitamins, antioxidants, iron, fiber, calcium and protein—at least artisanal

---

EAT YOUR CRUSTS

Remember how you used to eat your sandwiches from the middle, leaving the crusts on your plate? Remember how your parents would tell you to eat the crusts, because that's where the vitamins are? (Not that that ever really worked on you.) Remember when it dawned on you that your parents weren't making any sense, that all of the bread is made out of the same ingredients and so, nutritionally speaking, the insides and outsides should be the same?

Well, it turns out your parents were right: The crust *is* better for you. German researchers have discovered a cancer-fighting antioxidant amino acid (pronyl-lysine) in concentrations eight times higher in the crust than in the rest of the bread. As explained in the *Journal of Agricultural and Food Chemistry* in 2002, the process of baking bread creates this particular antioxidant, which is not present in unbaked dough. It *is* in wheat, rye, sourdough and quick breads, and especially in stuffing and bread pudding, or any dish where bread is broken into smaller pieces and baked—creating more bread surface area and, effectively, more crust. Darker breads like pumpernickel and whole wheat have more pronyl-lysine than does white bread, if you need any more reasons to switch from white bread.

---

breads do, particularly whole grain and sourdough breads. In fact, between 10 and 12% of wheat flour is protein. (Since not all breads are created equal, nutritionally speaking, see chapter 8 for more information on selecting the best breads, including specific brand recommendations.)

Poultry and Meat

For people who, like me, choose to eat meat, The Diet Code calls for including it in about half your protein selections, with the other half coming from vegetable sources. This won't be a precise split every day, but include animal protein (meat, eggs, fish) twice each day, and round it out with vegetable protein another two times (like beans or nut butter), with one more up for grabs: maybe make the fifth some cheese or yogurt.

You'll be perfectly fine, nutritionally speaking, without animal products at all, but if you do eat meat, be sure to choose vegetarian/ grass-fed, free-range, organic, antibiotic-free meat whenever possible. I don't buy into the Food Police crackdown on red meat. More than half the fat in beef is mono- or polyunsaturated, approved by nutritionists everywhere. And of the 46% that *is* saturated fat, about a third is made up of stearic acid, which does crucial work in the body, repairing cell damage. And anyway, there's no need to be afraid of a little saturated fat anyway, as explained in chapter 4. Beef also contains plenty of creatine, which is necessary for building muscle (which is why it is sold in pill form to bodybuilders). All meats and poultry are complete proteins, providing all the essential amino acids our bodies need but can't make on their own.

Eggs

Eggs are a very Italian food; Italians are more likely to have an egg on their plates than meat. Here's another food with a pointless bad reputation: The cholesterol in the yolks isn't going to raise your cholesterol level; it's excessive saturated fat that's going to do that. And eggs are naturally low in saturated fat and rich in protein, making them an excellent choice for anyone trying to build muscle and burn fat. And now in most grocery stores, and certainly in health food stores, you'll be able to find eggs from chickens fed a diet rich in essential fatty acids to produce eggs boasting high omega-3 levels. Even if you pay 3 dollars per dozen for quality eggs, that's still only 50 cents a serving (two eggs) for 12 grams of protein, making even the best eggs about the cheapest source of protein available.

Dairy Products

I use a lot less dairy than many people do, but when I do use it, I never choose nonfat varieties. They are by definition highly processed foods full of fillers, not to mention unnecessary carbs, and in a way

---

FERMENTATION AND WHY IT'S GOOD FOR FOOD

One of the best things to have in your food is bacteria. That statement depends on the kind of bacteria, of course, but I'm a big fan of lactobacilli in particular. Those little guys turn starches and sugars into lactic acid, and in the process improve the availability of nutrients, preserve food, predigest starches (lowering their glycemic indexes), produce antibiotic and anticarcinogenic byproducts and increase antioxidant values.

Furthermore, eating fermented food helps us digest all food: We rely on "good bacteria" in our guts to break down food so we

(continued on next page)

can absorb the nutrients therein. But modern American digestive tracts are drastically low in these probiotics (healthy intestinal flora). In addition, much widely available food is of compromised quality, with low levels of many nutrients to begin with. So we really need to get regular influx of the good bacteria from our food and to feed the desirable bacteria so they can do their job. Then we can absorb all the micronutrients we need. Without the assistance of good bacteria, the body doesn't recognize when it is satiated because it knows it still lacks nutrients. The less nourishing our food is, the more likely we are to overeat it. In overweight people, there's an excellent chance their bodies don't have enough of these probiotics and the digestive enzymes they create. That leads to overconsumption, as just described, as well as to bloating, gas, indigestion and constipation, among other woes.

Fortunately, there's a simple and delicious solution to this problem. Include food sources of probiotics in your diet: yogurt, kefir, artisanal cottage cheese (not commercially produced varieties), ricotta cheese, crème fraiche, sour cream, buttermilk, pickles and sauerkraut (made the old-fashioned [fermented] way), kimchi, miso, tempeh—and wine, beer and sourdough bread.

Many chutneys, relishes and condiments are traditionally made through fermentation as well. All soft, fresh cheeses used to be made this way, though you can't count on it nowadays— that's the same story for most of the dairy products listed above. The craft of making most of these fermented foods isn't easily industrialized, and modern commercial processing uses acetic acid or vinegar as poor substitutes for authentic fermentation. So you'll have to shop around a bit; look for labels that say the product includes active cultures or is "naturally fermented." You should be able to find yogurt like that easily and should be able to round up mascarpone, ricotta and cottage cheese made through fermentation at your health food store. Look for pickles, kraut and kimchi in the refrigerated section (*not* canned) made without vinegar or acetic acid—nothing much besides the vegetable, salt and perhaps some seasoning, like caraway seeds in kraut.

more dangerous than obvious fake foods because they appear to be something natural and are marketed as a *more* healthy option. Even low-fat dairy products can fall into this trap, so I'd just as soon enjoy the lusciousness of full-fat products. That includes butter; half a table-spoon, or a quarter-inch slice off a regular stick, is only 50 calories. Fermented dairy, like yogurt, kefir, cottage cheese, ricotta and crème fraiche, are your best bets in the dairy category; they help tune your intestinal tract for optimal digestion and absorption of nutrients.

The calcium dairy famously provides builds strong bones, and there's also evidence that it assists in weight loss, perhaps by increas-ing the breakdown of body fat and inhibiting the formation of new fat stores. Whatever the mechanism, a study done at the University of Tennessee concluded that dieters getting at least 1,200 milligrams of calcium daily (four Diet Code servings) lost almost twice as much as other participants getting less. Artisanal Italian cheeses like ricotta and Romano rank as the best calcium sources. Parmigiano Reggiano, for example, has 336 milligrams of calcium per ounce, about twice that of processed American cheese.

Fish

Fish is my personal favorite protein. Introduce a variety of fresh fish into your diet at least twice a week. Opt for the ocean run species (see the Fundamental Foods section); pick up any fresh local fillet at your market. Some of the recipes I've included in chapter 10 have been known to make fish lovers out of people who swore they didn't like fish. Sometimes, not liking a food means you've never had it prepared well.

A Diet Code pantry isn't complete without a few cans of tuna, sar-dines or smoked herring that will open into a meal in minutes. The common 3- to 3.5-ounce cans are perfect single-serving sizes. Work these into your diet once or twice a week. (A can of sardines alone supplies a full week's dose of omega-3 fatty acid, the weight loss fat.) I pick up a weekly treat of vacuum-packed smoked salmon, mackerel or trout for a Sunday antipasto brunch spread (see recipe on p. 212).

Olive Oil

Olive oil is a Diet Code essential because of its many beneficial properties as well as what it contributes to the taste and texture of food. It
lowers bad cholesterol and raises the good, helps you feel satisfied
after you eat and provides antioxidant protection—all the good things
monounsaturated fats do (see chapter 4).

Now that you can join olive-oil-of-the-month clubs or go to olive
oil tastings and watch blindfolded experts identify oils by region, the
issue is not so much *whether* to include olive oil in your diet, but *which*
olive oils to include. And really, that's a matter of personal taste. As
you develop a taste for olive oil, you may want to keep a few types on
hand, choosing the one you use according to what you're making:
strong tastes to stand up to meats, peppery oils to dip bread in, flow-
ery oils for salad and so on.

Of course, you'll want to choose quality oils, taking into account
color, aroma and taste. "Expensive" does not necessarily mean "best
quality"; nor does inexpensive mean an oil is inferior. As a baseline, a

---

BEST USES OF MEDITERRANEAN OILS

When exposed to heat, all oils start to break down and oxidize;
the temperature at which that begins to happen depends on the
oil. To make sure you get only health benefits from your good
oils, learn to use them at the appropriate temperatures.

- At high heat: grapeseed
- At medium heat: sunflower
- At low (or no) heat: olive, walnut, sesame
- Not for cooking (drizzle on afterward): flaxseed, pumpkin
  seed

good oil will be clear and not smell or taste rancid. Beyond that, the color, taste and smell that is best is the one you like.

Nuts and Seeds

Nuts and seeds are loaded with protein, fiber, good fats, vitamins (especially E) and trace minerals. Almonds provide calcium, for example, and walnuts are a great source of omega-3s. Research has shown that various types of nuts help reduce the risk of heart disease: A study at Harvard had volunteers trade 127 calories worth of other carbs for 1 ounce of nuts and found a 30% decrease in heart risk. Those who swapped nuts for an even amount of saturated fat saw the risk drop 45%. This worked even with peanuts, although they are technically legumes, not nuts.

WHAT YOU WON'T EAT

The Diet Code is a complete, balanced, satisfying and sane way to eat. It works because it includes all food groups rather than faddishly forbidding one or another. What it *does* cut out are highly processed, nonnutritive, manufactured "food" products. Leave most prepackaged

---

WATCH WHAT YOU DRINK

You need to watch what and how much you eat, for sure. We are a nation defined by consumption—nearly always overconsumption. But what you *really* need to watch is what you drink, especially sodas (even diet sodas), fruit juice, trendy coffee concoctions and alcohol, which can easily add hundreds of extra and empty calories to your daily intake.

(*continued on next page*)

• **Soda.** We've been downing it for a century, during which time the original 6- to 10-ounce bottles have morphed into super sizes ranging from twice the earlier maximum (20 ounces) to a full half-gallon (64 ounces)—often intended to serve just one person! That's between 65 and 200 grams of sugar (a sky-high glycemic load) and 250 to 800 calories just in what you're drinking. Diet soda may be lower in calories, but recent research suggests the artificial sweeteners may actually be making us fatter just the same.

• **Juice.** Commercial fruit juices and "nutribeverages" (sports drinks or juices with various nutritional supplements mixed in) rack up just about the same numbers as sodas, meaning equally bad news for your glycemic load. Some may give you vitamins or be spiked with added nutrients but can never compare to whole fruit for overall nutrition (fiber being a key component stripped out of juice). Furthermore, any benefits always come with a big dose of sugar.

• **Coffee.** It's been consumed by humans for over 500 years, and a good old cup of joe is only about 40 calories with cream. Cool. However, the new latte and frappe concoctions can pack 20 times that load—a whopping 800 calories for the average 20-ouncer. That's equivalent to *3 pounds* of cooked pasta with marinara sauce and parmesan cheese.

• **Alcohol.** Wine and beer in moderate amounts are beneficial to health. They are actually nutritious, too, containing microelements from the natural fermentation process (much like those found in bread or yogurt) and antioxidants. Hard liquor, on the other hand, is nonnutritive and much rougher on the body in general because the alcohol is so concentrated. The "toxic" in *intoxication* is no accident! You are much more likely to overconsume hard liquor. It's a lot of calories in one drink, too (even more so in a sugary concoction), especially considering that you don't get any nutrition in the bargain.

Smart choices include water, teas and broths, as discussed further in chapter 9.

items—especially those containing artificial colors, preservatives, sweeteners, sugar alcohols, starches and hydrogenated fats—out of the grocery cart. Don't stock up on soft drinks, fruit juices, commercial baked goods, chips, fatty deli meats or soy "meat" products. Limit or avoid refined sugars and deep fried foods along with denatured grains and fats.

THE DIET CODE
FUNDAMENTAL FOODS PYRAMID

I encapsulated this ideal dietary ratio in graphic form, creating The Diet Code Fundamental Foods Pyramid, drawing my inspiration from the Great Pyramid, with its 52-degree angle of slope rather than from the United States Department of Agriculture (USDA)'s much-maligned version. The result is a single structure based on ancient

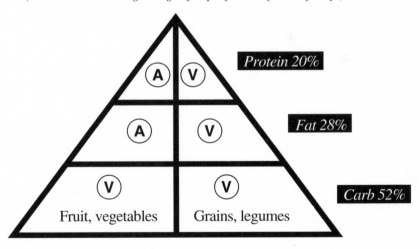

The Diet Code Fundamental Foods Pyramid
(Constructed with 52-degree angle of slope of Great Pyramid of Khufu)

Protein 20%

Fat 28%

Carb 52%

Fruit, vegetables   Grains, legumes

(A) *Animal Sources*
(V) *Vegetal Sources*

THE LORRAINE CROSS

In dividing three levels into two halves, The Diet Code Fundamental Foods Pyramid incorporates the two-armed cross that's come to be known as the Lorraine Cross. Originally used in Sumer (Mesopotamia) as an ideogram of egalitarian leadership, the design evolved as a symbol of tolerance and unity between the three related religions—Judaism, Christianity and Islam.

The king of Jerusalem granted the right to use the symbol to Godefroi de Boullion, duke of Lorraine, and it flew over his party carrying Hebraic and Islamic maths from Solomon's Temple to France, a watershed moment that ushered in the age of the Gothic cathedral.

In the early twentieth century, the Lorraine Cross was promoted as a universal appeal against the inhumanity of industrialization and the production of chemical warfare agents during World War I.

---

math, relating *duality* (animal and vegetable) to *trinity* (carb, protein and fat)—that is, relating the initial numbers in the Fibonacci sequence, 1, 2 and 3. In this way, my pyramid condenses the primary sources of optimal nutrition, encapsulating the secrets of a truly balanced diet.

The Diet Code Fundamental Foods Pyramid base represents the 52% of total calories that should come from Fundamental Carbohydrates: half vegetable and fruit, and half grains and beans—and including a bit of wine, beer and dark chocolate! (Almost all Fundamental Carbohydrates come from plant sources; animal sources, such as yogurt, cottage cheese, ricotta cheese, mascarpone, eggs and sausage, generally make up less than 2% of dietary carbs.)

The upper levels of the pyramid divide fundamental fats (28% of calories) and proteins (20% of calories) equally between animal sources (fish, eggs, poultry, beef, lamb, dairy products) and vegetable sources (nuts, seeds, olives, avocados) and their oils.

At face value, The Diet Code derives three-quarters of daily calories from plant and one-quarter from animal sources. It can be equally successful in vegetarian or even vegan versions, however. I do believe animal products are an important and beneficial part of a balanced diet, especially given diverse world populations and regional differences in environment, economics and food types available. But I don't think animal products are a necessity, and I know some people who retain full strength and vigor on an all-plant diet. I used to be vegan myself, eating no animal products or byproducts (even honey). This whittled my weight to about 20 pounds *below* where I've stabilized now. I was a bartender at the time, and I could still manhandle half-kegs of beer when I was working the weekend night shift.

But at this point in my life, I do like a good steak now and then. And I feel best with some animal protein and fat in my system. I realize some people thrive sans animal products, however, and many more avoid them for ethical or philosophical reasons; so I made sure The Diet Code could accommodate any dietary approach on the vegan-to-carnivore spectrum. Math, like music, is a universal language, so it creates a diet anyone can play.

Grounded in the best possible foods to eat, which you will learn to eat in ideal proportions, this plan feeds your body in harmony with its own design, in tune with the design of the entire universe. That's strong. That's beautiful. That's meant to last.

Chapter Six

The Principle Five

Life, if well spent, is long.

—Leonardo da Vinci

Inside every older person is a younger person wondering what the hell happened.

—Cora Harvey Armstrong

Scientific invention has outstripped our appreciation. We moderns fuss more about weight and health and length of years than humans ever have before. Supplements and surgeries, therapies and bio-technologies have advanced to satisfy both our needs and neuroses. They've also strapped us with a unique contemporary crisis: longevity. We spend a lot of energy worrying about our waistlines and choles-terol counts and blood pressure; but in the end, what we must face is how we've spent our time.

Leonardo goes so far as to define time in terms of *content*. Pack more living into your days, he infers, and your life will lengthen. Nanotechnology reshapes matter on an atomic level to engineer life extension, yet it is not more sophisticated than a mathematical re-statement of an observation made by Leonardo: A line enriched by a wrinkle, ripple or curve is longer than a straight one.

The Diet Code can be distilled to five—count 'em on your hand—principles for living. That's five adjustments to your eating habits and life in order to reach good health, a healthy weight and a life so rich you don't think to measure it in terms of years. And, as the years stack up, this handful of principles of good living won't leave you bewildered over what you've become.

As Franklin Roosevelt recognized, "Rules are not necessarily sacred; principles are," so instead of giving you rules just begging to be broken, here are five timeless principles for transformation:

1. Choose Fifteenth-Century Mediterranean Foods

✵

2. Just Two It

✵

3. Proportion Your Plate

✵

4. Speed Up

✵

5. Slow Down

PRINCIPLE #1: CHOOSE FIFTEENTH-CENTURY MEDITERRANEAN FOODS

Ask yourself, *What would Leonardo eat?* Choose those natural foods the original Renaissance man could have dined on, all of which would have been fresh, local, organic, seasonal and handmade. Basing each meal on these superior foods, known since Roman times as ideal for the human body, ensures you'll get everything your body needs for peak performance—and nothing you don't really want in your system.

Leonardo grew up in Vinci, one of the small villages dotting the steep, sunny hills around Florence. Those hillsides, crisscrossed with rivers and streams, were covered in low groves of silver-white olive trees and flowering almonds among the vertical black-green of cypresses. Garden plots surrounded those Tuscan villages, bringing forth a wealth of fruits and vegetables, among them asparagus, figs, fava beans, greens, garlic, squashes, pomegranates, onions, cucumbers, peaches, spinach, leeks, melons, cabbage, apples and artichokes. Grape vines, like garland, were often strung between trees. Orange, lemon, apricot and pear trees scented the air buzzing with bees, kept for pollination as much as for honey, and housed in golden domed baskets.

Villagers cultivated even the steepest land, building earth and stone terraces to protect against erosion of the rich soil and laying out neat, practical geometric fields as pleasing to mathematicians and painters as to farmers. Further toward the outskirts of towns like this lay fields of wheat and barley and pastureland. Every day heard the familiar bells of roaming sheep and goats (being raised for meat, milk and wool) and the pecking, scratching and gabbling of fowl (layers and roasters).

Later in Florence, Venice and Milan, Leonardo lived amidst over-flowing markets and street bazaars. Merchants plying Arab and Asian trade routes returned with sugar, spices, teas and coffee—exotic produce and flavors originating from Africa to the Far East intermingled with native fare. I imagine browsing street stalls in New York City's Chinatown to be about as close as you can get to experiencing what the glorious confusion of those old Italian markets must have been like.

Even in urban areas like these, there would be small farm plots on the outskirts of town and common green spaces called *vigna* (literally, vineyards) right in the city not only for public gatherings but also for growing fruit trees and vegetables and for raising small animals, like rabbits and chickens. In addition, the wealthiest brought with them the products of their rural landholdings to sell.

Seasonal

Last September, my oldest son desperately wanted a blueberry pie. So I sent a friend out for berries, and he returned with the requisite 6 cups—and a receipt for $17.94 for a quart and a half of berries from Chile. That's what was in the stores at peak blueberry season *in Maine*! So, too, a January peach today is shipped thousands of miles over untold days from wherever it really was in season—and where it was selected and grown more for the properties that allowed it to survive such a journey than for taste or nutrition. It's a hard, bland, mealy thing worth less than the memory of the bewitching, brandied essence of a luscious, orchard-picked fruit of late summer. (My pie, nonetheless, did turn out "wicked good." One thing I can do is bake!)

Of course, some foods could be stored against lean times in the long stretches between harvests, but most food during the Renaissance was eaten seasonally. Produce, obviously, was eaten as it ripened, but even meat varied in availability (and cost) throughout the year: Pigs were slaughtered in early winter; lambs were born in the spring; fish were prevalent during Lent, when eating meat was forbidden by the Catholic Church. Household staples that spanned the seasons included loaves and cheeses, olive oil, wine, nuts, pickled vegetables and dried fish.

It's a model we should still follow today. Food is tastiest in season and keeps the body tuned to the regional climate, decreasing our chances of catching colds and other infections. Determining just what *is* in season is something of a lost art, however, when pretty much anything you want is for sale all year round. Portland, Maine, at the same latitude as Florence, gives me a cheater's line to figuring the Tuscan cycle. I love my greens, so spring-to-winter, a rotation of spinach to chard to kale to cabbage would closely match Leonardo's fare. Cost is often a clue: Lower prices can be a rough guide to what's in season.

Local

Italians shop *nostrale*, buying "our kind." That is, they buy local produce and artisanal products made *all'occhio, cuore e mano* (with an eye, heart and hand for quality), hand-produced in small batches under direct human supervision. To do the same yourself, frequent local farmer's markets and small neighborhood stores offering handcrafted food. It's as good for the environment and the economy as it is for you. Supermarkets deliver convenience, and you can build Diet Code meals from what's available at chain stores—I'm not an advocate of "gourmet." But it's the small operations that create community—the "mom and pop" corner store, the neighborhood baker, the street vendor. And without community, we lose our humanity. Do your part: Shop as local as you can.

There's no comparing the taste and nutritional value of these products to anything industrially farmed or factory made, and the inherent satisfaction that comes from eating these foods means you'll naturally eat less without even being conscious of it. Organic, free-range and handmade foods may seem more expensive, but since you'll consume less, it won't really cost you any more. And, with most illnesses and diseases proven to be diet-related, eating this way is an investment in your health guaranteed to return monetary savings in health care.

Mediterranean

Research has repeatedly shown Mediterranean-style diets to be among the healthiest in the world. Mediterranean cooking is refreshingly low in starch, animal meat and fat, relying instead on fresh vegetables, beans, fruits and fish. It stresses simple ingredients—nutrient-dense Fundamental Foods proven through millennia to support natural weight control and optimal health.

Eating these foods in a simple balance of proportions will significantly increase the nutritive and metabolic power of your meals. Truly nourished and satisfied, your body can—and will—reach its own natural balance in terms of both health and weight.

The National Library of Medicine's journal database, PubMed, delivers almost 500 citations when you type in "Mediterranean diet." That's over 20 years of research, with 58 clinical trials looking at a way of eating that honors bread, pasta, wine, cheese, olive oil, vegetables, fruits, fish and fowl. So there's plenty of science available to

A PIZZA STORY

1000 BCE Etruscans in north central Italy bake *puls* (gruel cakes) seasoned with oil and herbs in hot ash.

500 BCE Greeks occupying southern Italy introduce the idea of using flat bread as an edible plate topped with eggs, onions, cheese, wine and spices.

75 CE Publicus Paquius Proculus of Pompeii purportedly parches the first *piza* (from Greek *picea*, describing a blackened crust).

100 CE Romans develop *placenta*, a wheat disc baked with cheese and honey.

1000 CE The word *pizza* first appears in a Latin codex.

1650 In Naples, *pizzaioli* (who underwent years of apprenticeship to earn the title "pizza maker"), baking in *laboratori*, create flat *sfizioza* that are folded and filled, making edible *libretti* (books). New Yorkers today still fold their pies.

1800 In Naples, the tomato is finally accepted as a topping; the word *pizza* is now common parlance.

1889 Don Raffaele Esposito creates the first tomato, cheese and basil pie for Queen Margherita di Savoia and King Umberto I of Naples: pizza Margherita.

1905 The legendary Gennaro Lombardi opens the first pizzeria in America at 53½ Spring Street, New York City (standing room only—no chairs!).

1924 Lombardi-trained Anthony Totonno opens his venerable shop in Coney Island, New York City. It is now the oldest pizzeria continuously operated and run by the same family in the United States.

1929 John Sasso, tutored by Lombardi, opens John's pizzeria on Bleecker Street in New York City, which is still turning out celebrated brick oven pizza today.

1930 The Lombardis add chairs to their establishment.

2004 The Italian Agriculture and Forestry Ministry announces strict new rules about what can be called traditional Neapolitan pizza, down to the type of flour, yeast, tomatoes and oil that can be used; how thick the crust can be and how hot the wood-fired ovens (and that it can only be prepared in wood-fired ovens) must get (905 degrees Fahrenheit). Forget "meat lover's specials," "salad pizzas" and even mushroom and pepperoni: Only marinara with garlic and oregano, margherita with basil and mozzarella cheese (from the southern Apennines) and extra-margherita with fresh tomatoes, basil and buffalo mozzarella (from Campania, the region in which you will find pizza's hometown of Naples)—qualify. Oh, and that pizza has to be a hand-formed round (no rolling pins) of no more than 14 inches in diameter.

back up claims about the wonders of eating a Mediterranean-style diet. I'll give you just a few recent examples of how powerful the effects can be.

Eating Mediterranean protects your heart, in part by lowering blood pressure and cholesterol. A study published in the *Journal of the American Medical Association* (*JAMA*) in 2004 by scientists in Naples followed patients with cardiovascular risk. Over the course of two and a half years, those who followed a Mediterranean diet compared to a "prudent" low-fat approach lost more than three times as much weight and significantly lowered a whole panel of scores indicating risk factors for heart disease. In fact, more than half of those patients got all their levels back into the normal range.

Experts estimate that following a Mediterranean diet could prevent up to 25% of cases of several common cancers. A study done in northern Italy of more than 22,000 patients called out the benefits of a higher consumption of fish, olive oil, vegetables, fruit and whole grain foods, and a lower consumption of red meat and refined grains. Results published in the *European Journal of Cancer Prevention* specifically linked a Mediterranean diet with decreased risk of several kinds of cancer.

Eating pizza even protects against heart attacks and some cancers, according to research conducted by Silvano Gallus and colleagues at the Mario Negri Institute of Pharmacological Research in Milan. Published in the *European Journal of Clinical Nutrition* in 2004, his results showed that people who ate pizza twice a week were less than half as likely to have a heart attack. Gallus reported in the *International Journal of Cancer* in 2003 that patients who reported eating the most pizza had the lowest risk of digestive tract cancers.

Overall, eating Mediterranean lets you live longer and be healthier along the way. Another study in *JAMA* in 2004 of over 2,300 Europeans, including Italians, between ages 70 and 90 looked at the effects of following a Mediterranean diet combined with an overall healthful lifestyle (nonsmoking, regular physical activity and moderate alcohol intake) and found the risk of death over a period of ten years to be cut in half when compared to the risk in participants not following those principles. Looking at diet alone, the risk of death dropped by almost a quarter. This and other studies call out particular health effects (heart disease, strokes, cancer) and consistently find benefits attributable to eating Mediterranean.

PRINCIPLE #2: JUST TWO IT

Arguably, the most important number for Italians is *duè*—two. Even Leonardo Pisano couldn't leave 1 alone and followed it fast with a partner in his Fibonacci sequence, which begins with 1, 1 . . . Italian culture, and especially Italian food culture, dismisses the solitary. As far as the Italians are concerned, everything needs a companion.

Italians can't even leave bread alone, hence the concept of companatico, or something to pair with the bread. It could be an egg poached in broth, fava bean paste, vinegared chicory greens, peppered oil or squid grilled at surfside. Apart from taste and appearance, remembering glycemic load (see chapter 4) secures the science in this. A little *fat, protein* or *citrus* reduces the GL of carbs (a boon for weight loss; see chapter 8), whether berries and cream, pineapple and yogurt, apples and cheese, spaghetti and meatballs, rice and ceviche (lime-marinated fish) or gemelli pasta with lemon juice. In each case, two is better than one. With The Diet Code program, you'll always pair a carb with a fat and/or a protein; this is one of the first actions of an Apprentice (see chapter 7).

In America, two things in proximity might incite comparison or competition, but for Italians, there's an escalation of energy between two things. That's *amore*—the start of love, where each grows a little in beauty in the reflection of the other. This is the core of Italian cooking, which does not so much reshape, rework or disguise foods as simply mate or pair them. The extraordinary results are, like bread or the Fibonacci spiral, greater than the sum of the parts.

So break bread together. Just as giving bread a partner (fat or protein) improves the way you metabolize it, sharing your meal improves your metabolism. Humans are by nature communal beings. Eating alone increases your chances of choosing quick-fix, unbalanced meals, gobbling food and overeating. Pair up, and the meal lightens on all fronts. While writing this book, some of the best meals I ate were simple affairs—pasta with anchovies, green olives, thick-rinded cheeses, smoked salmon, figs pressed in black pepper and wafer-thin slices of my sourdough wheat/rye/pumpkin seed bread— shared over wine with my friend Robert Gibbons, the poet, that melted into hours of conversation and supreme contentment.

PRINCIPLE #3: PROPORTION YOUR PLATE

Once you've chosen your Fundamental Foods from chapter 5 and paired them for potency, the next step is to combine them in proper proportions. As described in detail in chapter 7, you should design each meal and snack to create the Golden Proportion: 52% carbs, 20% protein and 28% fat; or, roughly, one-half carbs, one-fifth protein and one-third fat.

This is more or less how it would have worked out in the diet of the average Renaissance Italian: the majority of calories from carb sources, making full use of the bounty of vegetables and fruits grown in that climate, complemented with proteins and fats from both animal and plant sources. The five Fundamental Meals discussed on p. 109 will give you an idea of what the Golden Proportion will look like as you put it into practice.

The social inequalities that were part of Renaissance society were marked, in part, by food. It was peasant fare that formed something close to the Fundamental Foods Pyramid, like Leonardo's meal of bread, cheese and soup, or an omelet served with greens dressed liberally with olive oil and a little vinegar and salt. Dishes like these were popular across all social strata. The main dietary differences at the tables of the wealthy had to do with the extras they could afford. Because they were relatively expensive items, the rich ate more white bread, meat and sugar. Pasta, which was three times the price of bread, didn't become an everyday menu item until the 1600s (where that trend first took root in Naples), so Leonardo would have known it more as an occasional treat.

Renaissance Italians struck a wonderful balance in their sources of protein and fat through a combination of preference, affordability and the dictates of the Roman Catholic Church. Overall consumption of meat peaked at the time due to general prosperity and a relatively low population that could afford to devote more land to grazing animals than to growing grain. Still, meat was more expensive than grains and vegetables and even other sources of animal protein (eggs and cheese), so amounts were limited, except for the rich. The democratic pursuit of hunting produced lean game, like rabbit, and the lighter meat of birds.

The "bean-eaters" nickname was well earned, however, as people throughout the Tuscan area loved lentils, peas and chickpeas and derived a good deal of their protein from them. Almonds, too, were readily available and frequently eaten. And while Leonardo avoided meat for much of his life, most other people abstained frequently themselves to follow the dictates of the church, which forbade eating meat on regular fast days (three times a week), through the 40 days of Lent and on the eve of various religious festivals throughout the year. Fish was the usual replacement and was widely enjoyed.

Eggs were a staple of most households, and dairy mostly meant cheese, as milk spoiled too easily. Cheese, on the other hand, was made during the summer in the mountains, and some kinds—hard and dry forms—kept all year. Italians then, as now, enjoyed a staggering variety of cheeses: in curds and formed, soft and hard, fresh and aged, mild and rich, moist and dry.

Animal proteins were a source of fat as well, of course, but much of the fat in the Renaissance diet in Italy came from olive oil from the abundant olive trees across the countryside and, thanks in large part to the religious calendar, from fish. Olive oil was a mainstay—the fat of choice for most cooking—and quality oil was revered like fine wine.

I've chosen five Fundamental Meals that represent the taster's choice of the simple Renaissance foods outlined above: grains, greens, eggs, fish, poultry (game), beans and fermented dairy. These five meals compose a core dietary program unto itself—this is lifelong good nutrition distilled into just five plates. Check chapter 10 for actual preparation and portion size, but lock these Fundamental Meals into your weekly menu, and you'll be "Golden"!

Five Fundamental Meals

1) Porridge / Yogurt / Fruit

This ancient carb-rich combination is perfect for firing your metabolism in the morning as breakfast or for building muscle after a workout. Adding dairy and fruit to whole grains is age-old wisdom handed down in the form of traditional foods in societies around the globe. We now know that this strategy also serves to form complete protein and ensure good mineral absorption.

2) Roman Fish Soup

Besides being a perfectly balanced dish of salmon, kale, beans and leeks, the dish takes less than 15 minutes to prepare, start to finish! Vary the fish, even substitute chicken or sausage, and experiment with different vegetables and beans, and you have a simple dish you'll never outgrow.

3) Polenta and Greens with Eggs

This is the most requested plate on Sophia's menu: peasant food I've rescaled to a quick 4-minute cook time. There's no excuse for eating poorly anymore! You can substitute tempeh for eggs and beans for polenta. That last combination—*erbazzone e fagioli,* or greens and beans—is our second most popular dish, served accented with a little Grana Padano cheese.

4) Baker's Lunch

This is my standard fare: artisan peasant bread or a whole meal sourdough slice with cheese and/or white anchovies, or spread with nut or seed butter (sunflower, peanut, sesame-tahini or hemp). It's a great snack and perfect as a preworkout energy source, an economical answer to all those sports/nutrition bars. And to think it's just what my grandfather showed me 35 years ago.

5) Alla Cacciatore

This literally means "in a hunter's style" and is a classic Italian way to serve game: braised in tomato sauce. It doesn't have to be rabbit or pigeon—chicken is hard to beat. This slow-cook one-pot method transforms tougher, cheaper cuts of meat into melt-in-your-mouth delicacies, and the pot can be stocked with the vegetables of your choice: peppers, onions, greens, carrots, turnips etc. The carb can be polenta, pasta, bread, potatoes or rice. Whatever the mix, you'll spend a peasant's wage to dine like royalty.

PRINCIPLE #4: SPEED UP

When it comes to reaching and maintaining your ideal weight, your metabolism (the rate at which you burn calories) is your best friend or your worst enemy. A speedy metabolism burns off calories quickly and efficiently, before they get stored as fat. A sluggish metabolism stands by while what you eat is methodically packed away in fat cells all over your body. Once you know how to choose your foods, increasing your metabolism is your best bet for losing weight and keeping it off. The very best way to increase your metabolism is to exercise (though not necessarily in the way you think).

Metabolism, the body's use of energy, has three components: what's needed to keep your body's most basic functions up and running, what's needed to digest what you eat, and what's needed to fuel activity. You have more influence on and can reap more benefits from some of these than from others, so you need to know the difference.

First, your basal metabolic rate (BMR)—baseline, or resting metabolism—accounts for 55–75% of the calories you burn every day running your body's vital functions, like breathing. This is the first and, when it comes to weight loss, most effective of two ways exercise speeds up metabolism: by building muscle. Muscle is "metabolically active," burning calories even while at rest. Muscle cells always burn more calories than fat cells do. Your BMR increases in direct proportion to growth of your muscle mass but decreases with greater body fat.

Next, 5–15% of the energy your body expends each day is through the thermic effect of food (TEF), or the process of digesting your food. Diet, rather than exercise, carries the lead in increasing this form of metabolism. The higher the ratio of carb to fat in your food, the higher the metabolic rate is, because it takes more energy for the body to store carbs as fat than it does to store fat directly. That's thanks to the second law of thermodynamics, which states that converting energy from one form to another requires energy. Storing dietary fat as fat requires no conversion and burns essentially no calories at all. And complex carbs have half the calories (by weight) of fat, effectively giving them a head start in the metabolic process anyway. Furthermore, eating, in and of itself, expends energy.

Using Φ^3 to proportion your carbs and fats (or, roughly twice [1.86] as many carb calories as fat calories) will maximize this kind of metabolism. Eating smaller but more frequent meals that combine protein and carbs helps, too.

The third type of metabolism is what scientists call the effect of physical activity (EPA)—how much energy the body uses in completing daily activities. This is 20–40% of your total metabolism. Obviously, this is the second place exercise can really make a difference. EPA is much higher in active people than in the classic American couch potato. The more physical activity you do throughout the day, the higher your EPA. Your EPA also increases with the intensity, duration and frequency of activity. Exercise also improves your insulin sensitivity and the body's ability to process carbs. Keeping blood sugar on an even keel is another key to maintaining a healthy weight.

As it stands, lack of physical exercise means most Americans have very slow metabolisms. Women's metabolisms are typically slower than those of men (in part due to their lower muscle mass), and their bodies can be even more prone to storing food as fat. Even in the best-case scenario, metabolism is going to decline with age. In fact, it's slowing down from infancy on! Most of the calories babies take in are given over to the brain and internal organs, the body tissues with the most dramatic metabolic demands. As people grow through childhood and into adulthood, body fat increases and metabolism slows. Metabolic rate shoots up to see the body through adolescence (as you know if you've ever needed to keep a refrigerator stocked for a teenager) but slows again once full growth is achieved. There it stays until midlife, when hormonal shifts lead to decreases in muscle, further slowing the metabolic rate and causing the famous middle-age spread.

This is why so many people get away with careless eating and little or no exercise into early adulthood—and why it catches up with everybody in the end. Fortunately, regular exercise and a little attention to what and how you eat can counteract the downshifting of metabolic rate.

Yet one-quarter of all Americans don't get any exercise at all. Less than a third get 30 minutes a day, the minimum recommendation in the new government guidelines on nutrition, a standard set only to lower risk of chronic disease. For most people, losing weight will require more. Experts estimate that 300,000 Americans die each year from the effects of insufficient exercise. No wonder: Americans spend nine times more time parked in front of the television than they do at all exercise and physical leisure activities combined and put in more time driving a car than they do exercising. Many of us live in sprawling suburbs not conducive to using walking as a means of transportation or even just as entertainment or exercise. We practically live in our cars! We seem very attached to stationary electronic screens of various kinds and have gotten so desperate as to count throwing a Frisbee or carrying a load of laundry to the basement as physical activity.

Exercise can reset the "set point" the body uses to regulate weight, especially in conjunction with the metabolically powerful Fundamental Foods listed in chapter 5. Set point is that stubborn plateau our bodies hit when we try to greatly alter our weight. This effect occurs not only in weight loss, but, as bodybuilders know, in weight *gain* as well. So, speed up your metabolism with increased exercise and select foods, but have patience with your body as it changes gears or shifts its set point. From neutral to fifth gear is, after all, five distinct steps!

Exercise keeps muscles, tendons, joints and ligaments strong and flexible. It helps move toxins out of the body and supplies plenty of oxygen to all tissues. With exercise, you feel better and look better. You improve your sleep and your mood. You have more energy. Government guidelines published in 2005 promise benefits from exercise including "health, psychological well-being and a healthy body weight." Anyone who doesn't exercise is bound to accumulate excess baggage in at least one—and probably all—of those areas.

It doesn't have to be any particular form of exercise as long as it builds muscle, and it doesn't have to be any formal or organized program. You might like tennis, or swimming, or yoga, or weightlifting, or dancing, or you might just live a very active life. To stay healthy, move your body every day. Even follow the only specific exercise recommendation I'm going to make here: walk. Walking is simple, uncomplicated, variable and accessible to just about everyone.

Though I now get most of my exercise doing martial arts (and before that I lifted weights at the gym), I once perfected my own program of walking. I dropped 58 pounds doing it, too, in conjunction with a carb-rich, meatless diet. Inspired by the physique of bread-loving, town-hating nineteenth-century naturalist trekker John Muir, I footed it everywhere. I even sold my truck. From my own experience, I learned that a walking stick—a body-length staff alternated side to side now and then—was all that was needed to keep fit and muscular, including my arms and shoulders.

I love Ellen DeGeneres's line: "My grandmother started walking 5 miles a day when she was 60. She's 97 now and we don't know where the hell she is." Joking aside, walking 5 miles a day would be an excellent way to live to be 97. An ultimate exercise program, that would be about an hour and a half on your feet. A commitment like that will totally renovate your life. Even just an hour a day, walking nonstop at whatever pace is comfortable for you, would be a revolution. The actual American average is about a quarter of a mile each day. (Globally, the daily average is closer to 10 miles a day.) Start with less if you need to, and work up to it. But walk an hour a day, every day, for one solid month, and I guarantee you'll see results.

Skip the treadmill and do your walking outside as often as you possibly can. Look around. Engage the world around you. Walking outside is a wonderful way to tune into the rhythms of life, just like eating seasonal foods. Here again you can take a tip from Italy where, from Leonardo's time to now, people walk the city streets and country lanes *a spasso* (for pleasure). They are doing more than "getting some exercise"; they are enjoying themselves, meeting friends and enlivening their neighborhoods. Walking is not something apart from life that must be endured and then checked off the To Do list.

More Ways to Speed Up

Breathe deep. Just like fire can't burn in a sealed box and the carburetor on a car's engine controls the rate at which the gasoline can burn, oxygen affects our metabolism and the way we burn food. Advanced practitioners of yoga or the martial arts can alter their strength, endurance and need for food and sleep to miraculous degrees by varying breathing and oxygen intake. Just becoming aware of breathing and relearning to breathe with the belly instead of the chest (observe how a baby breathes) will further aid health and weight control.

Spice it up. Spicy food increases your heart rate and, with it, your metabolism. Enjoy hot peppers and other spicy foods often—slather your breakfast eggs with hot salsa, spike your black bean chili with cayenne or spread horseradish on a meat sandwich.

Stimulate it. Make use of another common stimulant to speed up your metabolism: caffeine. Avail yourself of green, black and white teas often, or coffee or espresso once a day, or enjoy an occasional treat of dark chocolate (½–1 ounce).

Challenge your mind and body. Pick up the pace of your walk or workout: Metabolism revs and revels with increased exercise intensity. Take up a foreign language, do a crossword puzzle or watch a foreign movie: Verbal and linguistic challenges are known to spark the brain and burn more calories. Difficult music does it, too. "Now's the Time" to check out the jazz musicians Charlie Parker, John Coltrane or Pharaoh Sanders or classical mindbenders like Béla Bartók, Iannis Xenakis or Thomas Adès. Or take in an abstract art exhibit. Even break out the crayons or paints yourself! Take up a hobby or physical activity that involves both sides of your body (and therefore both sides of your brain), be it juggling or knitting or playing piano. Even

learning to love unfamiliar foods gives your body and brain an immediate jumpstart and pays dividends forever after. Take, for example, developing a taste for cruciferous vegetables. Cabbage, kale,
cauliflower, broccoli, Brussels sprouts, collards and the like so often
challenge the American palate, until we learn to prepare them *al
Italiano*—braised al dente with garlic and olive oil, for example. Even
better are the ancient preparations of these veggies fermented to increase probiotic digestive enzymes, such as sauerkraut and kimchi.

PRINCIPLE #5: SLOW DOWN

Here's the yin for the yang above: While you are working to speed up
your metabolism, you should seek to slow down the speed of life in
other important ways. Americans approach food with such anxiety—
the dark side of our eternal quest for the perfect diet as the fountain
of youth—and with our speedy pace. In a better world, we would all
eat like Italians, enjoying our food, indulging our senses, sharing—
and loitering over—our meals.

One of the things that attracts me to bread making is the way it
inherently forces me into a slower pace. Dough won't be hurried. You
can't rush the rising of the dough or the firing of the oven—at least
not if you want to end up with bread worth eating. It can take an
entire day to make a loaf of bread; even, as with Phi Bread (see recipe
on p. 273), an entire week. That puts you in sync with the natural
rhythms of the world—or at least slows you down enough so you can
take note of them.

It was this same ideal of a slower pace of life and what it meant for
what and how we eat that Carlo Petrini took to heart in 1986 when he
opposed McDonald's opening in Piazza Spagna in Rome. He could
see that his country's distinctive regional cuisine and food traditions
were at risk, a scenario repeated countless times around the globe as
fast food chains and supermarket homogenization threatened to
dilute the power of quality food and authentic culinary traditions. He
couldn't stand by silently. Food production was becoming industrial-

ized, which produced cheap food but at a high cost to both environment and culture. The food supply was being standardized, tastes were being synthesized, farmland was being degraded, the experience of eating itself was being cheapened—and fast food symbolized it all.

Petrini's protests spawned Slow Food, a nonprofit educational organization currently active in 50 countries, with a total membership of over 80,000. Slow Food is on a mission to protect, promote and celebrate food heritage and traditions and the diversity of the earth's bounty. Slow Food rests on twin supports of food appreciation and environmental consciousness. The Tuscan-born movement advocates organic foods and farming; sustainable agriculture and biodiversity; small-scale food specialists and local producers; seasonal and local foods; heirloom produce varieties and animal breeds; and artisanal products like handmade bread, farmhouse cheeses, and wine and beer crafted by hand. Such foods, created with taste and tradition given primacy, form a core cultural identity, and protecting them also protects the communities that produce and depend on them.

Slow Food's American mission statement declares its focus on "reviving the pleasures of the table, . . . using our taste buds as our guides." We move so quickly through life today that we tend to forget the senses are important tools of knowledge. Slow Food appeals to that inherent wisdom, appreciating food as "a perishable art, as pleasurable in its way as a sculpture by Michelangelo or a painting by Titian. Not mere nourishment to be wolfed down, but culture to be savored."

Slow Food promotes "pure sensual pleasures, to be taken with slow and prolonged enjoyment." It stands for slowing down to achieve pleasure and quality in everyday life, first and foremost by honoring the convivial traditions of the table. Eating is a communal experience; food is better when it is shared. Any given meal, whether it's a simple sandwich or a multicourse repast, is best enjoyed with good company.

That's the way it was done in Leonardo's time. In *Daily Life in Renaissance Italy*, the historians Elizabeth S. Cohen and Thomas V. Cohen describe the social aspects of even the most basic meals: ". . . Men stopped together in the evening for a pitcher of wine; a woman supped on artichokes at her sister's house.... At home, on the benches in front of shops, at a tavern, people liked to eat and drink with friends and family. Indeed, these shared activities ... marked a human bond. They reinforced old ties and forged new ones. We have a word for this phenomenon, *commensality,* whose Latin roots mean 'sharing a table.' Those who do so are *companions;* the word itself once meant 'sharers of bread.'"

Italians today maintain the primacy of commensality. Family meals are a sacred ritual, providing a time for conversation and bonding. Friends are just as likely to gather around the table, joining the family or making a family of their own. It's just how I remember it being in my family growing up, with my nona hosting parties for 50 or more. No matter how many gathered from how many far-flung spots, the parties always had the feeling of family. Nona would line up about four picnic tables, end to end, to accommodate the 30-foot feast. All through the afternoon and into the night, platters of food would appear—and disappear! The homemade wine flowed. It seemed no one ever wanted to leave.

Dining together or alone, Italians take their own sweet time eating a meal. It's a part of the culture there, to the extent that many businesses shut down mid-day, the better to enjoy a relaxed lunch. Real food—whole, fresh, delicious—you wouldn't want to bolt down. Gobbling robs you of pleasure or forces you to chase pleasure by eating more and more, beyond reasonable hunger, just to lengthen the experience. Yet it is just this style we Americans specialize in, thoroughly trained by fast food ideals and eating-on-the-run habits.

For the first five years, I only opened Sophia's four days a week. To answer those asking for hours more like those in the rest of our 24/7 world, I posted the following anecdote in the entryway of Sophia's. It's an old story, passed by word of mouth and probably originating in India, and it sparked almost as much excited commentary in my shop as did the bread. It must speak to something even Westerners find resonating deep inside them, perhaps a vital piece missing from our "diet":

A visitor to a foreign land watched for some time as an itinerant craftsman hammered away on a delicate metal plate. "How much for this piece?" he finally inquired.

The worker tapped and thought, and eventually replied, "Ten coins."

"Hmm . . ." said the visitor, "and how much for ten such pieces?"

The metalsmith tapped on, then said, "Fifteen coins each."

"Fifteen?" asked the visitor, puzzled. "What if I were to contract you for a hundred of the same piece?"

"For a hundred, the price would be twenty-five coins each," leveled the artisan.

"Extraordinary!" blurted the flushed visitor. "By what system of reckoning do you establish such prices?" he demanded.

Soon the answer came: "To make one plate is for me a pleasure. To assign myself to a hundred would begin to rob me of my joy. The cost rises on one side because the cost rises on the other," said the artisan. "It is only just."

We are so far out of practice with eating leisurely meals that we need it broken down for us: Take small bites, savor each one, chew thoroughly, finish chewing and swallowing one bite before taking another and stop when you are satisfied. *Eat* when you are eating; don't watch TV or multitask at mealtimes. By the same token, don't habitually add eating to your routine when what you're really doing is sitting down to watch a show, going for a walk or phoning an old friend. Eating slowly allows you to recognize your body's signaling when it is full and to respond accordingly. And eating slowly is a prerequisite for eating mindfully. Be conscious of your food and your experience of it rather than just shoveling it in.

Eating slowly, with obvious enjoyment in the company of friends and family, plays a key role in keeping Italians slim—twice as many Americans are overweight as Italians, according to a *New York Times* column by Giuliano Hazan, written from Verona. Hazan points out two other ingredients in the successful formula—eating smaller portions and leading less sedentary lives—and emphasizes that it's not

THE PERFECT PEAR

I learned how to eat a pear from my grandfather. One hot August day when I was only three or four, I watched him cut hay by hand with a scythe, listening to the distinctive whooshing sound, feeling the sun bearing down and breathing air thick with chaff. When he took a break, he sat me down in the shade of a pear tree, picked up a fallen fruit, and pulled out a well-worn, curved pruning knife. He then carefully pared off thin slices and offered them to me on the blade of the knife. I can still taste the cool, sweet juice and remember the sure and practiced movements of my grandfather's rough workingman's hands. I felt like a king served like that, sheltered by the tree and by his company. It was a proper way to treat the fruit as well, savoring each delicate piece, quenching the thirst of both body and spirit.

any one food group that makes us fat, but rather our relationship with food and our lifestyles, concluding that how we eat is just as important as what we eat.

In a column in the *Boston Globe,* Lawrence Lindner reviewed government nutrition recommendations from around the world in honor of the United States' new food pyramid. While Britain's first rule (just ahead of "More fiber, less fat") is "Enjoy your food," Norway officially advises its citizens that "food and joy equal health," and Vietnam recommends choosing food "that is delicious . . . and served with affection," the United States has no place for pleasure in its rendition. Ten years ago when the pyramid was revamped (as it is legally required to be periodically), the committee in charge rejected the inclusion of the phrase "enjoy a variety of foods." It was thought that would encourage people to eat as much as they wanted indiscriminately. And that was the last time the notion of enjoyment was heard in that quarter.

Our culture provides all kinds of messages about food, from cooking techniques to table manners to acceptable food selections. (Do "we" eat snails? goat? squid?) Italy has a culture and tradition of enjoying food with moderation built in—a baseline assumption rather than a psychologically more difficult restriction. Here we choose volume over quality, overeating in a vain attempt to make up for lack of taste and nutrition. We tend to look at food as an entity just waiting to make us fat or sick, then scarf huge quantities nonetheless, creating guilt. We choose our foods by numbers (fat grams, carb counts etc.) rather than by taste or tradition. Food—choosing it, preparing it, eating it—becomes just another stress.

We imbue food with the powers of salvation and damnation; we seem to think if we could just eat correctly, we could live forever—but if we slip up, we will be punished harshly. A study of cultural attitudes toward food done by a University of Pennsylvania psychologist and a French sociologist turned up this delectable nugget, as summarized by Michael Pollan in an article in the *New York Times Magazine*: "Americans associated food with health the most and pleasure the least. Asked what comes to mind upon hearing the phrase 'chocolate cake,' Americans were more apt to say 'guilt,' while the French said 'celebration'; 'heavy cream' elicited 'unhealthy' . . . and 'whipped' from those groups." Americans worried more about food and reported less pleasure from eating than the French, Japanese and Belgian people also surveyed. (The study didn't include Italians, but you can guess where they stand in the land that gave us gelato.)

If we eat a slice of birthday cake, we're likely to say we've been "bad" or that we were "tempted," as if it really were the devil's food. We seem to expect some kind of medal for self-denial, accepting thinness as a form of moral superiority. And just where does that leave the humans among us, imperfect, pleasure-seeking mortals that we are? Fortunately, reframing the issues frees us from the saints and sinners view of what we put into our mouths and leaves us free to both enjoy our food and live at our ideal weights.

Our national episodic obsession with one diet trend or another reflects not any real advances in nutritional understanding, but our anxiety about what to eat and why. Perhaps we have too many food choices available to us and no intrinsic way to winnow them down. We fall sway to one passing diet guru after another—irrespective of the quality of their information—as if the next one will finally solve the riddle for us once and for all. Yet no pat answer ever lets us relax. In Italy, they just keep eating as they have for generations, guided by tradition and taste, following long-established habits inextricably linked to their sense of who they are and where they come from. According to a 2004 article in *National Geographic,* Dr. Atkins's books have sold many millions of copies in 25 languages around the world, but it's never been rendered in Italian. Coincidence? I don't think so. The Italian way of eating is a *fad*-free diet, and it's the only bandwagon truly worth jumping on.

We must leave behind the anxiety that permeates our American attitude toward food in favor of a more Italian approach, reveling in food as a source of pleasure and well-being rather than fearing it. As Virginia Woolf put it, "One cannot think well, love well, sleep well, if one has not dined well."

Chapter Seven

The Diet Code Program: Apprentice, Journeyman, Master

Myth is the secret opening through which the inexhaustible energies of the cosmos pour into human cultural manifestation. Religions, philosophies, arts, the social forms of primitive and historic man, prime discoveries in science and technology, the very dreams that blister sleep, boil up from the basic, magic ring of myth.

—Joseph Campbell, from the prologue to
The Hero with a Thousand Faces

Order and simplification are the first steps toward the mastery of a subject—the actual enemy is the unknown.

—Thomas Mann

The Diet Code program follows a unique learning curve that sets it apart from other diet programs just as distinctly as does its choice of foods and the way it combines them. The typical diet program sets you up for failure from the beginning simply because of the way it is structured. As with anything else, good design is crucial. And here once again, the best design is the one most in tune with human bodies and human ways of being. Human experience isn't linear; it runs in a curve (like phi). The three-part program laid out in this chapter bends to fit just right.

Following the arced path of the classical trades, The Diet Code program is divided into three phases: Apprentice, Journeyman and

Master. The initial phase is somewhat simplified to allow you to incorporate these strategies into your life in manageable increments. Like any fine craftsperson, you're building something meant to last, and that can't be rushed. You need the right materials and the right tools—and you need to know how to use them both well. Focus now on choosing the right foods in the right portions and eating them in close to proper proportions, and you'll start shedding extra pounds right away.

You'll refine and intensify your approach in the second phase, increasing your results as you increase your precision. If the first phase didn't bring you to your ideal weight (and it might well have), this one will. You'll work with an eye more on details as you develop a real feel for your craft.

The third and final phase really isn't programmatic at all; rather, it marks your complete integration of this way of eating. If you persevere to this level, the whole process will become intuitive. You won't be doing The Diet Code; you'll be *living* The Diet Code, and its principles will come naturally to you without a lot of conscious effort. You'll be at your ideal weight and you'll stay there, because once you've cracked The Code, you'll never be without the answer.

The opening chapters of this book have given you an understanding of the principles put to use in this chapter, and the next three chapters give you the nuts and bolts you need to get started, taking you through stocking your pantry, planning your meals and cooking Diet Code dishes. This chapter, then, gives you the road map so you can see clearly the route that lies before you and recognize the landmarks along the way.

In a 1987 PBS series with Bill Moyers, the famous mythologist Joseph Campbell explained how he distilled a comparison of crosscultural legends into a universal pattern he called the hero's journey. Each myth—all myths—are "always . . . one shape-shifting yet marvelously constant story," according to Campbell, and create a three-part motif: "the call" (departure), "the ordeal" (initiation) and "the mastery of worlds" (return). This is the standard and only guide that serves to validate our experiences, Campbell maintained, and he saw understanding this as a vehicle for personal transformation. It's an answer to a universal longing.

The Diet Code program is designed to tap into the same core truths that give our myths and legends their power to move us, a power that holds across time and cultures. Myths and legends permeate the richest and most enduring parts of human existence; they inhabit and inform our lives to this day. We never tire of them, as demonstrated by the massive appeal of such modern iterations as *Star Wars, Lord of the Rings* and *Harry Potter,* because they are not just hazy, mystical figures from the past, but rather comprise a vital blueprint for contemporary living. The Diet Code leads you to your natural and healthy weight by framing the way you eat as a mythic journey. This is your Grail quest, your turn to bear the ring.

Typical diets fail us because they have us choose an end instead of an experience. Diets also fail by making the beginning the most important. Conventional diets impose the fanfare of greatest change at the start, while the learning thins out as we continue. We lose interest and snap back like a rubber band. By doing what no business would do—giving entry-level employees rather than seasoned veterans high-level tasks—these diets force the issue, making us take it all on at the start, so we inevitably crash the program. These diets proceed according to a linear structure utterly at odds with the normal growth curve of everyday life. In today's world, it isn't just when it comes to diets that we tend to rush and shorten experience. Charles Lamb quipped about this modern malaise: "I always arrive late at the office, but I make up for it by leaving early." I see this inclination not as a sign of our true nature but as a reflection of the degree to which we are out of touch with our own mythology.

In the interest of following the form most suited to those of us on the journey, The Diet Code, like Campbell's template, is bowed, or hill-shaped. In fitting our lives so naturally—the same way The Diet Code foods fit our bodies—the program allows for weight loss that happens just as naturally. Since you will be feeding your body what it really needs in order to lose weight rather than depriving it, and since what you will be feeding it is delicious (not "diet") food, and comfort food at that, your body will automatically reach for its own best balance without it feeling like a lot of effort from you. The one great secret of weight loss is . . . to eat! The pounds will come off, yes. You will reach your ideal weight, but it won't feel like a struggle or a burden. In other words, The Diet Code doesn't really feel like what you've come to think of as a diet at all. And it is certainly not meant to be the time-limited experience most diets are. The Diet Code is for *life*.

Which makes it, after all, the only true diet, in the original sense of the word we've since warped to have quite different connotations. The ancient Greek root of the word diet, *diaitasthai*, means leading a life or selecting a way of life. A diet is—*should be*—a way of choosing, selecting and shaping your body and life, not some quick-fix, temporary approach. Choices become habits and become *you*. That's The Diet Code in a nutshell: Apprentice (making the choices), Journeyman (setting the habits), Master (being you).

Diet, then, can be used to lose, maintain or gain weight, but all in the continuance of life. Meal skipping and food denial (forms of starvation) and junk food and fad diets (forms of malnutrition) oppose life: They are not and can never be real diets. They will disrupt metabolism, leading to rebound weight gain and overall poor health. The Diet Code powerfully activates metabolism, permanently reshapes the body and allows you to be fit and trim for life.

Most weight loss plans—and all the trendy ones—hype you into believing they cause the loss of fat (adipose tissue), while in reality they produce any transitory success through water loss (dehydration) and breakdown of muscle and organ tissue (catabolism). True fat loss only occurs at a rate of up to 8 to 10 pounds per month, about 2 to 2.5 pounds per week, and that's just what The Diet Code offers. Any regimen that strips weight faster than this will disrupt normal metabolic function, not only ultimately failing, regardless of any initial appearance of success, but also adversely affecting health and vitality in the process. I don't care what they're calling it—any drastic weight loss plan is just a repackaging of the oldest forms of weight loss: malnutrition and starvation. The Diet Code won't—*can't*—promise unreasonably fast weight loss. What it does promise is *healthy, permanent* weight loss with an ease you may never have thought possible.

APPRENTICE

A mythic journey begins amidst the familiar. An urge to change, always some form of self-enhancement or self-improvement (like improved health or weight loss), impels the first steps. A *herald,* in Campbell's terms, brings the hero a call to adventure. The call is whatever makes you bolt upright and want something different—whether a career change or a loss of 10 pounds. Campbell also identifies a *mentor* as a necessary guide for a hero—an Apprentice—early on, allowing the development of confidence in a new or alternate world.

Judging by the fact that you are reading this book, you've heard your call. Or, perhaps this book *is* your call. Either way, welcome to the path. I hope you'll allow me, through the book, to be the mentor guiding you through the early part of your journey.

Apprentice-at-a-Glance

Everyone begins The Diet Code as an Apprentice. Those of you who feel the temptation to plunge straight into the more complex Journeyman program should resist it. Its greater complexity will feel like a natural transition to the experienced Apprentice, but starting the more involved phase as a novice will set you up for failure. You'd be biting off more than you can chew. This is not a race; there's no clock ticking toward a deadline. You don't need to be satisfied with the numbers you see on the scale in X weeks. It's true that Journeymen can expect faster results, if that's the strategy they choose, but that's only sustainable for people fine-tuning their approach, not for people overhauling it.

Beginning at the beginning, then, your first task is to get used to using the basic components of The Diet Code in their simplest form: to reach and maintain your ideal weight and optimal health, choose the right foods (Fundamental Foods), and increase their power by eating them in the correction portions and proportions. A big part of your job is simply to get used to eating whole foods and how they taste and feel in your body.

You will start to lose weight as soon as you implement these basic changes to your diet. Your metabolism will respond right away to the true nutrition you are now providing your body with, thrumming to life to power your body with maximal efficiency *for life*. This Apprentice stage alone may well be enough for you to reach your ideal weight and stay there. Even if you never go any further in The Diet Code program, your health will certainly improve, and your weight will stabilize. For many people, the Apprentice plan *is* The Diet Code.

The key points for an Apprentice are explained in full in this section but are summarized here for quick reference:

#1: Eat five meals a day. Eat frequently to provide your body with constant fuel, charge your metabolism and avoid hunger pangs. Plan three main meals a day and two minimeals—snacks or appetizers.

#2: Use correct serving sizes. Use the guides here to make sure you put an appropriate amount of food on your plate.

#3: Combine Fundamental Foods. Make the best pairings—and threesomes—of each of five food groups to keep your blood sugar stable and set the stage for steady weight loss.

#4: Approximate the Golden Ratio 1–2–3. Create the relationship between serving sizes of the different food groups that maintains a natural balance of macronutrients. Start with the appropriate amount of a grain food, add twice as much (by weight) of a protein food, and add three times as much (as grain) vegetable and/or fruit.

#5: Take a day off. On one day each week, eat *whatever you want*. The Diet Code is not about deprivation, and no diet that is will ultimately work. Everybody needs to blow off a little steam now and then, so there's an escape valve built right into the program.

$3 + 2 = 5$

The first change for most people adopting The Diet Code is to eat more—at least, to eat more frequently: five meals a day. The Diet Code includes snacking—encourages snacking—but *planned* snacking. Grabbing something to eat just because it is in front of you or because you haven't eaten in too long leads to making bad choices. You end up eating a bag of chips rather than yogurt and granola or a gummy energy bar instead of fresh vegetables with hummus.

So as an Apprentice, you'll have three main meals each day—a fairly traditional breakfast, lunch and dinner—and two small meals or snacks. Here, you'll get some general strategies about what, specifically, all those meals should include. Then check out chapter 9 for specifics—a series of sample menus specially geared to the Apprentice to guide and inspire you.

The Five *Food Groups*

In preparation for creating meals out of Fundamental Foods and in Golden Ratio proportions, let me introduce you to the *five* food groups: Grains, Vegetables and Fruits, and a trio of proteins: Fatty Proteins (richer in fat than in protein), Lean Protein (richer in protein than in fat) and Starchy Protein (protein foods rich in carbohydrates)—henceforth to be known in Diet Code shorthand as G, VF, FP, LP and SP, respectively. The subdivision of proteins may seem a little confusing at first, but if you stop to think about it, you probably already know for the most part which foods fall into which categories:

G (grains): bread, pasta, whole grains, whole cereals
VF (vegetables and fruits)
FP (fatty protein): cheese, nuts, seeds, nut butter, olives, avocados

LP (lean protein): fish, poultry, meat, tempeh, eggs, cottage cheese

SP (starchy protein): potatoes, beans, peas, corn, yogurt

Serving Sizes

The first step for the Apprentice learning to assemble Diet Code meals is learning to bypass the super-size portions that have come to seem normal, even at home, in favor of more sensible servings. The guides below will help reorient you. You may be shocked at first when you realize the relationship between what you've been dishing up for yourself and what you should actually be eating, and the right size may at first strike you as a bit paltry. But don't worry. I've seen it over and over again: When you choose nutrient-dense foods and eat them in the right combinations and proportions, the recommended serving sizes will satisfy you. There's no going hungry on The Diet Code.

When you move on to the Journeyman stage, you'll be measuring out your portions, but for now, make it easier on yourself by estimating. Below you'll find the sizes you should be aiming for; then further along you'll find a "hand-y" reference you'll always have with you to help you check that your servings are appropriately sized. Obviously, I can't give you the serving size for each and every food—and even if I did, it wouldn't be really useful to you unless you memorized them—so these are general guidelines.

The specific foods I've included here I chose because they are some of the most important ones on The Diet Code, and they'll keep coming up as you lay out Diet Code meals.

You'll have to keep in mind that there can be quite a range of foods within these groupings—1½ cups of spinach salad is a different thing altogether from 1½ cups cooked spinach—so unless and until you are ready to begin weighing your food (see the Journeyman section), employ a "fudge factor" here and some common sense. If you buy a 1-pound package of cheese, you get 16 1-ounce servings out of it. Is that 1⁄16 of the brick you just set alongside your crackers? If you buy a

APPRENTICE
DIET CODE SERVING SIZES

Food Group	Serving Size
FP: *Fatty Protein* olives cheese nuts, seeds, nut butter avocado ricotta	1 oz (8–10 olives) 1 oz 1 oz (2 tbsp nut butter, ¼ c whole nuts) 2 oz (¼ fruit) 2 oz (¼ c)
G: *Grains* pasta, crackers, whole grains, bread, cereal, rice, polenta Bavarian-style bread	2 oz (⅓ c) dry; 4–8 oz (⅔–1 c) cooked depending on the grain or the noodle 2 oz (1 ⅜-inch-wide, 4-inch-square slice)
LP: *Lean Protein* cottage cheese fish, poultry eggs tempeh steak	4 oz (½ c) 4 oz (½ c) 2 (large) 4 oz 4 oz
VF: *Vegetables and Fruits* most vegetables winter squash most fresh fruit most dried fruit	6 oz (1½ c) 6 oz (1 c) 6 oz fresh (1 c) 1½ oz dried (¼ c)
SP: *Starchy Protein* yogurt potato beans	8 oz (1 c) 8 oz (1 c) 8 oz (1 c)

WHAT IS 2 OUNCES OF BREAD?

Two ½-inch-thick slices from a multigrain sandwich loaf
(standard 4- by 4½-inch size)
One 3⅓-inch section from a rustic baguette
One ⅜-inch-thick slice from a Bavarian-style bread (standard
4-inch square)
Two 6-inch sprouted grain tortillas, like Ezekiel 4:9 brand

pound of steak, that's enough to serve four people (4-ounce servings). A pound of pasta will cook up enough to feed eight. The main idea is to reality-check yourself. Most people have a good idea about how much 1 cup holds but don't pay much attention to how that relates to the mound of pasta in front of them. An Apprentice pays attention.

Hand-y Measurements

One of the best tools for gauging appropriate serving sizes is a tool you are always carrying with you, right at the end of your arm.

Our earliest measurements were based on the human body; today's unit of measurement the foot is an obvious relic of that. The earliest applications of the Golden Ratio sprang from this bodymath (see appendix B). Leonardo's most recognizable study of the subject revolved around a human body scaled in Egyptian cubit measure derived from the human hand. His *Vitruvian Man* was sketched precisely to show the Golden Ratio as revealed in the human form. And now your body, specifically your hand, provides you with the initial measures you need to follow The Diet Code. An apprentice in any trade, from stonecutter to violinmaker to baker to magician, needs simple, hands-on confidence. Using your own hand as a guide to portion size guarantees yours.

Use your *thumb* to size up rich foods, like cheese and nut butters.
Use *four fingers* to size up a slice of bread.

Use your *cupped hand* to measure dry whole grains, like rice, oatmeal or bulgur; or snack foods like nuts, chips and dried fruit.

Use your *palm* to gauge proteins, like meat, fish, tempeh and (whole) eggs.

Use your *fist* to measure fruits and vegetables; potatoes, beans or yogurt; or cooked pasta or rice.

You'll note this hand-y system inherently adjusts serving size according to body size. Bigger people will naturally need slightly bigger portions.

These measurement guidelines ensure portion control and also proportion. Just as your fingers and hand go together in graceful proportion (Golden Ratio proportion, in fact), so too do the foods measured out according to them. As you learn to make Diet Code combinations of Fundamental Foods, these are the amounts called for to balance macronutrients, provide adequate fuel and nutrition and support weight loss.

READ THE LABEL

Here's one secret of The Diet Code: What you need to know about serving sizes is often already there on the label. There's nothing special about Diet Code serving sizes. They certainly diverge from what too many of us have habitually come to dish out, but they're right on target with what the USDA and responsible nutritionists everywhere have been recommending for years. So any packaged food—and there are good ones, even as you get much pickier about using only whole foods—will tell you right on it how much you should eat of it and how many portions that particular package is meant to provide. In most cases, those bits of information will line right up with Diet Code recommendations.

THE EYE OF HORUS

Horus, the Egyptian god of grain, is represented by a falcon-headed human figure. The eye of Horus is a familiar hieroglyph, a human eye with the cheek markings of a falcon and, in the ancient Egyptian system of measurement, a representation of a system of fractions used to measure parts of a whole. Five millennia ago, the Egyptians had already laid out a pattern that corresponds with Diet Code serving sizes.

The whole eye represented 1 *heqat* (almost 5 liters, or a bit over 1 gallon)—a standard grain measure. The eye hieroglyph is composed of five parts representing the five senses, plus a sixth, the eyebrow, indicating the highest sense—mind or thought. Each part of the eye is carefully scaled to represent a particular portion of a heqat. Its smallest unit, five *ro,* stood for "that which feeds one mouth" and is about Φ^2 (2.6 ounces or ⅓ cup)—The Diet Code portion size for grain! (See appendix B for more on the mystical relation of numbers 5 and 6.)

The Clean Plate Club

Here's a tip for Apprentices: *Don't serve family style.* Make it a habit to fill your plate with what you (now) know are the correct servings sizes, and there's your meal. No more, no less. (Go ahead, join the clean plate club—as long as it's always a Diet Code plate!) It's much harder to tell what an appropriate serving size is when you're scooping it out of a huge full bowl. Those serving bowls are just going to mean an extra layer of dirty dishes to clean up anyway!

In addition, randomly going back for seconds (easily in reach, family style) drastically changes your serving size, of course, but it also throws everything out of proportion (more on that in a moment). If you've served yourself properly in the first place, you really won't need seconds. Properly combined and proportioned Diet Code meals will satisfy you. Most of us rush to put more on our plates before we've really finished with "firsts"—and we probably rushed through those firsts, too. If you take time to eat mindfully, appreciating what you have while you have it, and give your body some time to take in and register that it's eaten a full meal, you'll notice your body stops sending hunger signals, and you'll naturally be ready to stop eating. In the bolt-your-food style prevalent in America today, there's no time for your body to know it's been fed before you are overfeeding it. That's exactly why so many of us eat way too much without ever really knowing that's what we're doing. Given a chance, our bodies will tell us they've had enough.

For the same reasons, it's a good idea to prepare only what you're planning to eat/serve at that meal. Everyone eats their intended share—without worrying about seconds or leftovers. Diet Code meals are generally so quick to prepare that it's not really much of a time savings to double any given recipe so there will be automatic leftovers ready for a second meal. All too often, what really happens is that everyone eats more than they would otherwise, and your planned leftovers don't end up being enough to make another meal. If you really prefer to cook extra and/or to serve family style, my advice would be to put only enough for that meal into the serving bowl and to store away the rest even before sitting down to eat. Divided into serving-size containers, those leftovers are already pro-portioned for whoever ends up reheating them. And everyone at the table will have a clear idea of their fair share of what is served.

The Power of Pairs

To begin to find the proper proportion in your diet, remember Principle #2 ("Just Two It") and start pairing foods so that their joint benefit to your body is greater than either alone. The key advantage of doing so is the reduction of glycemic load, as discussed in chapter 4. This is the power of many classic couples from around the world—

bread and cheese, fruit and nuts, beans and rice. *Si sposa,* they are called in Italian culinary dialect, essentially "marriages" of foods. (Italians are big on flavor marriages, too, as in the duos orange and fennel, tomato and basil, polenta and sage, and coffee and chocolate.) You'll make full use of this strategy in designing your two daily small meals.

You can pair any two foods from any two of the five food groups to create your minimeals. The only thing you *don't* want to do is double up on rich carbohydrate sources at a single meal; pick potato *or* corn on the cob *or* pasta *or* bread *or* rice *or* other grain *or* wine *or* beer. There is an exception to this exception: yogurt or beans combined with cereals, grains or pasta create complementary proteins, the benefits of which outweigh the concern over a few extra carbs. But in general, choose one high-carb food at a time. Watch out for the starchy proteins in particular so they don't sneak up on you.

To give you the general idea, *all* the possible group combinations, with example foods, appear below. It's almost a week's worth of food ideas but is intended for you to use as a springboard in identifying your own favorite duos. You'll find a lot more inspiration in the menu plans in chapter 9.

Finally, I want to call attention to the fact that the power of two doesn't end with the glycemic index. Foods are best paired anyway, the same way a meal is best shared. Creating a rudimentary union of two disparate elements puts bow to fiddle. It's only when two are together that music begins.

As The Diet Code unfolds, you'll learn more exacting and sophisticated ways to create the ideal proportion of macronutrients. For now you can rely on nature's wisdom to give you much of what you need just by using the power of two. Any one type of food typically contains a significant proportion of another, the way nuts have protein and fat or beans have protein and carbs. As you may have deduced from the arrangement of the five food groups, this is particularly the case when it comes to protein foods. Most proteins are also major sources of fat. Carbs may also carry fat and/or protein. Protein and fat tend to occur naturally together in foods in roughly the proportion you'd want them in; you can ensure that by properly pairing

FOOD DUOS				
Food Group			**Food Group**	
FP	peanut butter	+	whole meal bread	**G**
FP	olives	+	tuna	**LP**
FP	cheese	+	apple	**VP**
FP	avocado	+	black beans	**SP**
G	brown rice	+	chicken	**LP**
G	polenta	+	Swiss chard	**VF**
G	granola	+	yogurt	**SP**
LP	salmon	+	artichoke hearts	**VF**
LP	sirloin tips	+	corn on the cob	**SP**
VF	onions	+	peas	**SP**

The last combination may seem less of a meal to modern sensibilities, which see onions as a seasoning or garnish, but accurately reflects the prominence they had in the diets of old, which they still deserve today. Onions and peas were an entire meal for Italian peasants. In the time of Charlemagne, laborers were given the daily ration of 1 pound of the vegetable bulb to 2 pounds of bread.

foods from different groups together. In this way, two becomes three: Pairing two foods gives you all three macronutrients.

From Duo to Trio

Three is just as powerful a number in The Diet Code as two. To create your three larger main meals a day, you'll need to pull foods from three food groups. We'll soon get to how these trios (and duos) create the Golden Ratio, but for now we're just concerning ourselves with making the most of three-ness.

Moving from duos to trios obviously allows for more variety in

FOOD TRIOS

(FP) ricotta	+	**(G)** pasta	+	**(LP)** shrimp
(G) bulgur	+	**(LP)** egg	+	**(VF)** zucchini
(LP) turkey	+	**(VF)** kale	+	**(SP)** potato
(SP) beans	+	**(FP)** cheese	+	**(G)** tortilla
(VF) peaches	+	**(SP)** yogurt	+	**(FP)** hazelnuts
(G) bread	+	**(VF)** wine	+	**(FP)** cheese

taste and texture in each meal. Variety keeps you from getting bored and ensures a regular supply of the full compliment of nutrients. But while it opens these doors, it also, usefully, closes some others. Thinking in threes will keep you from going overboard, the way typical American menus do, by putting multiple vegetables on the plate or by representing every food group at every meal. Life is complicated enough as it is; there's no need for elaborate meal planning to add to the chaos. This restraint, typical of Italian cooking in general and mine in particular, will keep you focused on Fundamental Foods in

EAT BREAKFAST

Starting the day with a healthy meal will boost your metabolism. This is the best time of day to have carb-rich foods like cereals, granola, porridge, whole grain toast or muffin, yogurt or bananas— properly combined with a fat or protein, of course. Studies show that people who eat breakfast naturally spread out their calorie intake more evenly over the course of the day, which not only keeps you properly fueled but also lets your body burn calories efficiently. Harvard Medical School researchers studied thousands of Americans and found that those who ate breakfast every day were far less likely to be obese than were those who skipped it.

desirable portions and proportions. It's also the secret to meals that can be made in a flash.

Elbert Hubbard declared, "Every man is a damn fool for at least five minutes a day; wisdom consists of not exceeding the limits." When you do establish limits, wonderfully clever variations come together within

---

THE TRINITY

The power of three has long been lauded in multiple fields of human endeavor. The notion that three elements combine into a more potent whole undergirds art, architecture, engineering, social dynamics, religion and the artisan baker's code, among others.

Three-sided forms are renowned for their stability. From hewn knee braces on timber-framed houses to the open air angle trusses of the Eiffel Tower, the triangle is unshakeable. The oldest freestanding structures on earth, the 5,000-year-old pyramids on the Egyptian plain of Giza, are testament to the architectural durability of the triad. And, of course, the idea of a trinity looms powerfully in religion as well as in architecture. Roman dictate created the theological Holy Trinity in the fourth century CE, at the time of the emperor Constantine.

But a sacred trinity of foods—bread, wine and cheese—predated Constantine by tens of centuries. From the age of Leonardo back to the time of Charlemagne and further still to Alexander the Great and even pharaonic Egypt, these three foods stood together, a timeless dietary core.

The earth abounds in natural foods eaten in their natural states that formed the basis of primitive diets: seeds, nuts, fruits, roots, bulbs, leaves and land and sea animals. The trinity are "supernatural"—alchemical foods that require human intervention, created for people by the work of people. Together these foods provide both the stability of architectural triangles and the inherent spirituality of trinities, which accounts for their lasting value throughout the ages.

them. On p. 138, I show some examples that cluster Fundamental Nutrients in wise combinations. The prep tips in chapter 8, menu plans in chapter 9 and recipes in chapter 10 will give you many more ideas about how to pick and prepare all these Fundamental Foods.

The Golden Proportion

The next important idea for an Apprentice is the basic proportions of the duos and trios of Fundamental Foods on your plate. Where a Journeyman will actually weigh or measure food portions, as you'll soon see, an Apprentice estimates ideal serving sizes. The simplest way to create a Golden Ratio of macronutrients at every meal is to start with a grain (G) in the recommended serving size stated right on the package. Taking pasta as an example, that would be 2 ounces (dry), which cooks up to about 6 ounces, or anywhere between ⅔ and 1 cup, depending on the noodle. (You could also begin with the serving size noted on the hand-y chart.) Then, choose twice as much (by weight) of lean protein (LP). To continue our example, let's say you are in the mood for chicken with your pasta. You should have 4 ounces of it. Complete the meal with three times as much vegetable or fruit (VF) as grain. For our hypothetical meal, let's make it asparagus—6 ounces worth (1 cup).

For most food group combinations, this one-two-three approach will roughly approximate the 52% *of calories* from carbs, 28% from fat and 20% from protein that represents the Golden Ratio (which we'll get to more specifically in the Journeyman section). The ratio will be reached through the combination of the carbohydrates in vegetables, fruits and starchy proteins and the natural balance of fat and protein in so many foods (assuming you're using full-fat products rather than pale imitations). You might not hit the Golden Ratio at every meal when you are estimating this way, but averaging them all together, you will have an overall Golden Ratio diet. In addition, your estimating skills will improve over time, bringing you closer and closer to exact proportions.

The meal plans in chapter 9 provide plenty of prearranged options for you to choose from, so you can always be sure you're hitting the Golden Ratio by following them.

Your Sweet Tooth

One great thing The Diet Code will give you that no other plan really does is dessert. Real desserts, not some chemical mess full of artificial sugars and fats that never really satisfies anyway. Sometimes you might choose to top off a meal European style, with fruit, cheese or nuts, but you'll also be able to enjoy a piece of rich chocolate cake or your favorite pie.

This is a diet of inclusion—there are no real foods you have to say goodbye to forever. Doing so is a setup for failure anyway, both physiologically and psychologically. Restrictive diets make you feel like you have less, and it's human nature to compensate by craving more. The secret of The Diet Code is knowing you can have everything—in proportion.

Making that work simply means paying attention to substitutive balance. If you want biscotti for dessert, just have a salad or vegetables with your grilled chicken and skip the side of rice at that meal. Eat that raspberry truffle, but don't have the potato.

The Diet Code flexes this way just as it does to accommodate the inclusion of wine or beer for those who enjoy having a drink with dinner. As long as you keep the ratio right, treating yourself this way occasionally won't disrupt your health or weight at all. Some sweets are easier to swap in than others, it's true, but there's never anything you'll have to do completely without.

So you'll find a range of desserts in the recipe section, ranging from Sophia's indulgent flourless chocolate cake to a Sardinian confection of almonds, honey and orange peel. You'll learn some traditional Italian baking techniques that were originally devised to conserve expensive flour and dairy but also turn out to be more healthful, like using ground nuts, nut paste or olive oil.

Your Day Off

Eating whatever you want one day a week is more than just a license to indulge. As long as you eat The Diet Code way for six days each week, you can pick one day to eat *whatever you feel like* without compromising your overall results. Indulge if that's what you want to do; for an Apprentice, the seventh day is usually host to at least a little dietary rebellion. You may be surprised to find that if you nourish yourself well with whole foods and can count on a time for treats without regard for their caloric profile, your cravings for unhealthy foods begin to dissipate.

This seventh day should also serve as a day of reflection—a day to get you thinking about the food choices you make, where you are on your journey and how your body feels after eating different kinds of foods.

Checking in with yourself regularly like this is the best way to know whether and when to move on from the Apprentice phase. The basic guidelines laid out earlier will provide you with a balanced and nutritious diet that will have you well on your way to reaching ideal weight. You'll be reaping the full health benefits of the Fundamental Foods, and your weight will be stabilizing at or close to what's healthy for you. Your cravings will be reduced. You'll be fitter, whether or not you've gotten where you wanted regarding your weight. If you have gotten to your ideal weight or can at least clearly see your destination, perhaps you'll be content to stay right there. Feeling good about yourself and your body is far more important than whether you are carrying an extra 10 pounds. Your pace of progress on The Diet Code depends on your metabolism, how much exercise you get and how poorly you were eating before, among other things. (The worse your original diet, the greater the shift to The Diet Code and the faster the weight will come off.) If you're not satisfied with your success or have reached a plateau you want to push past more quickly, or if you simply want to engage more deeply with and more closely control what you eat, it may be time to become a Journeyman.

At the very least, you should not move on until you are thoroughly comfortable enacting the Apprentice principles. There's no gain in moving ahead before you're really on top of your game here. Give yourself plenty of time at the Apprentice stage to get your new habits really ingrained in your life (which may take months). Only then are you ready—and even then, only if you *want* to be ready—for the increased challenges of the Journeyman.

JOURNEYMAN

A journeyman endeavors to extend and hone the artisan's eye, heart and hand through the tradesman's accumulation of day-to-day doing. In one of the old trades, for example, the apprentice went from being the one who was made to work the bellows and watch to the journeyman who was entrusted with the hammer and worked the steel. In the framework of Campbell's mythic journey, this is the stage of initiation in which the hero must pass the "guardians of the threshold" into the unknown. Little helpers or omens along the road may guide the hero, but as any tradesman knows, there is no longer a benevolent or paternal master or mentor. The Journeyman level is all about "breaking through personal limitations," as Campbell would have it. You'll be honing your technique, improving your fluency and speeding your weight loss.

For those who pursue the Journeyman stage of The Diet Code, this is going to mean more work than was required of an Apprentice. The Journeyman phase is for those who like the details and those up for a challenge—but also those who want more or different rewards. As a Journeyman, you'll lose weight more regularly and quickly than you did as an Apprentice. If you haven't already reached your ideal weight as an Apprentice, the Journeyman phase will get you there. As you control your food intake more precisely, you'll also be able to calibrate your results more precisely, firing up your metabolism even more or dropping weight more quickly, if that's what you decide to do, or fitting The Diet Code more closely to your own life, or striking the best balance between diet and exercise in your quest for good health.

As a Journeyman, you'll orchestrate mathematically precise and satisfyingly delicious meals. Just as Leonardo demonstrated that synthesis is possible between science and aesthetics, the Journeyman's task is to move beyond simple meal planning to unite measure and meaning, math and emotion, rule and savor to create a diet that is more precise and therefore more able to deliver consistent, predictable controllable results. Still, though, it is rooted in hard and fast numbers and aims to develop in you a more sophisticated feel for food and your relationship with it. Continuing The Diet Code journey in this way is within the reach of anyone who wants to learn it. The Journeyman stage requires more effort and more control, but in the service of increased flexibility. Ultimately, the Journeyman will be finding freedom in The Diet Code, not more restrictions. The hard work of the Journeyman is meant to prepare you for breaking through to the Master level, in which living and eating this way no longer seems like an effort at all.

Journeyman-at-a-Glance

The key Diet Code points for a Journeyman are explained in full in this section but are summarized here for quick reference:

#1: Eat six meals a day. You'll be eating a bit smaller and a bit denser than you were as an Apprentice, spreading your calories out over six rather than five meals—three main meals and three minimeals.

#2: Count your calories. The best way to give your body the fuel it needs without excess destined to be stored as fat is to know just how much fuel that is. Here you'll learn how to tell how many calories you need to take in in order to lose, maintain or even gain weight, depending on your goals. Find the number that's right for you to guide you as your prepare your menus and meals (with additional specific guidance to be found in chapters 9 and 10).

#3: Balance your food groups. Each day you should get (at least) two servings of food from Grains (G), two from Lean Protein (LP), two from starchy protein (SP), three from Fatty Protein (FP) and five from Vegetables and Fruits (VF).

#4: Measure your food to create the Golden Ratio. Pull together #2 and #3 by actually measuring out desired serving sizes—for an excellent relative balance of macronutrients *and* the number of calories appropriate for your body.

#5: Have a day of rest. Just as you did as an Apprentice, eat smart for six days, and dance with the devil for one.

$3 + 3 = 6$

As a Journeyman, you'll eat six times a day, spreading out your intake more evenly throughout the day to more evenly (and powerfully) stoke your metabolism. Each of your three main meals and three minimeals will be a bit smaller than they were previously, though the total amount of food you eat will remain roughly the same. For your three main meals, choose one food from each of any three groups (make a trio); for your three snacks, choose one food from each of two groups (make a duo) or make it a (wisely chosen) single.

You can arrange the timing of the different-size meals however suits you. Keep it the same every day or vary it, whichever way you like. Have a minimeal for breakfast if you want to or a main meal midafternoon, if that suits your schedule. Use a minimeal as an appetizer course to dinner or as a dessert. Or shift dessert until a couple hours after the main meal and eat it as a snack. Part of the point of putting in all the work at the Journeyman level is so you can sculpt the program to your individual needs and preferences. Journeymen get to know the rules so well that they know exactly how to bend them without breaking them.

Calories Count

To successfully control your weight, you need to deal with calories. You *don't* need to fixate on them or research or memorize the exact counts in every food you eat. But you *do* need a general awareness of them, starting with how many your body needs. If you take in more than that, you get fat. That's the bottom line. No amount of hocus-pocus on behalf of any diet theory can sidestep this fact, no matter what other gimmicks try to shift your focus or promise results without counting calories. You certainly don't have to tally every single one you come into direct contact with, but neither can you blithely ignore them. Not if you want to reach and maintain your ideal weight.

A calorie is simply a measure of the energy food stores—the food's "potential energy." (Technically, 1 calorie is the amount of energy or heat it takes to raise the temperature of 1 gram of water 1 degree Celsius.) Carbohydrates and protein have 4 calories per gram, and fats have more than twice that (9 calories per gram). Different foods are metabolized differently, so calories are not all the same in the effect they have on the body. Whole foods contribute less to weight gain and more to good metabolism than the caloric equivalent of processed foods. Besides that, for 250 calories, you can have a 1.5-ounce candy bar you'll wolf down in a couple bites or a 6-ounce grilled chicken breast, or a ¾-pound dish of pasta with fresh marinara sauce and parmesan cheese. Your choice.

Theoretically, broccoli will make you as fat as shortening, given sufficient (and outrageous) amounts. Looking at it from the other side, though, butter might make you less fat than oil, if you use them in equal serving sizes. Butter has more volume than vegetable oils, so there are fewer calories per tablespoon (65 in a tablespoon of whipped butter, versus 120 in a tablespoon of oil). A low-fat or low-carb brownie will still pack a wallop in the calorie department (not to mention artificial ingredients galore) and contribute every bit as much to your waistline as any other brownie. What all this *really* means is that it is easy to manipulate perceptions with calorie-speak.

So much depends on how you look at it. That's why so many of us were duped into accepting that a bowl of oatmeal or a slice of bread could make us fatter than a bacon cheeseburger served sans bun.

Target Practice

Before we get to how many calories are in your food, I'm going to take you through determining how many calories should go into your body. Here's how to figure out your target intake: Take your target weight—the weight you want to stabilize at—and multiply it by 15.

And there you have it. Want to weigh 130 pounds? Regardless of what you weigh right now, aim for 1,950 calories a day (130 × 15). Is 160 pounds more realistic for you? Get 2,400 calories a day (160 × 15).

In real life, there are variables complicating this simplistic equation, of course, among them your activity level and the idiosyncrasies of your particular metabolism. In this section, I'll break all that down for you and show you how to tailor a target calorie count just for you, based on your target weight, current weight and height.

Recall for a moment what was discussed in chapter 6 about your basal metabolic rate, or BMR. No matter what your weight, it takes about 10 calories per pound per day to maintain body functions. That is, a 160-pound person requires about 1,600 calories a day for basic survival and organ maintenance—essentially, just to stay alive.

Of course, in real life, people's calorie needs exceed that, depending on how their individual bodies run and how active they are. On average, an active body needs closer to 15 calories per pound to maintain (neither gain nor lose) body weight. That 160-pound person realistically uses about 2,400 calories a day. The greater the physical (and mental!) strain, the greater the need for fuel. So if the theoretical 160-pound person is an Olympic swimmer, he or she might consume as many as 5,000 calories a day. On the other hand, if the person has a desk job and is otherwise a total couch potato, taking in even half the swimmer's calories would cause him or her to pack on some pounds.

To determine *your* caloric need so you can adjust your daily intake accordingly, you want to be realistic, both in terms of what your body needs to run and what a reasonable target weight is for you. Getting too few calories can be as harmful as getting too many—excessively low caloric intake *stalls* weight loss and injures the body. On The Diet Code, you identify your target weight, then aim for the number of calories each day to maintain that weight. So, if you currently weigh more than is good for you, you're going to stop eating the daily calories that support your current weight and instead eat the daily calories appropriate for the weight you want to get to.

The method given here sets you on the path for a sane weight loss of a pound or two a week, 4–8 pounds a month, by diet alone. Increasing exercise will naturally add to weight loss and is of course the preferred way to go for all kinds of health reasons. (Adjust your caloric intake, however, if the combination makes you lose weight faster than this desirable rate—anything dropped that speedily is destined to come back on, and probably sooner rather than later.) So the system flexes to account for varying activity levels.

Making sure to look at your situation clearly, here's how you set your goals:

- Choose your target body weight—the weight you *want to* be, or what is reasonable for your height. The Metropolitan Life height and weight charts suggest that, on average, for women, weight should be roughly twice height. So a 5-foot, 5-inch woman should be shooting for around 130 pounds (2×65 inches). Men's weight should be approximately 2.3 times their height—this 5-foot, 10-inch baker, for example, should target around 160 pounds $(2.3 \times 70) = 161$.
- To find out how many calories you need to eat to maintain that weight, multiply it by 15. Continuing with the example above of a 160-pound man, he'd need 2,400 calories a day to stay at that weight.

Looking at it another way, if our hypothetical man weighs more than 160 pounds right now, he's been taking in more than 2,400 calories. Say he weighs 185 at the moment. He's probably been munching

---

EXERCISE

Adopting any reasonable but steady exercise regimen will kick-start your weight loss better than any other single thing. Obviously, it will help in any phase, but if you didn't take up something as an Apprentice, it's time to rethink it now and consider, as a Journeyman, increasing your commitment in this way.

My advice about exercise is twofold and brief. One: Just do it, whatever it is, however you do it, wherever it gets done. The details matter little as long as you move your body on a regular basis. And two: Do whatever you enjoy. That's what you'll keep doing, rather than abandoning it as the steam runs out of whatever transient enthusiasm got you going.

Personally, I practice martial arts about three times a week, for about an hour (a very intense hour) each time. That's in addition to the hard labor of being an artisan baker. As a general target for everyone, I recommend three hours a week—half an hour a day every day, with one day off a week—but no more than six hours a week (unless you're at semiprofessional athlete status).

---

on about 2,775 calories a day to maintain that weight. His basal metabolic rate dictates he needs 1,600 calories a day essentially to stay alive; he needs 800 more (or 2,400) to sustain a normally active life—but he's taking in 375 calories more than that each and every day. It takes 3,500 extra calories to add a pound of fat onto your frame, so our hypothetical man could gain a pound in less than ten days.

Now let's say our 160-pound person is a woman leading a relatively sedentary life and wishing to slim down to about 130. She'd have to drop her daily calories to 1,950 (130 × 15), rather than the 2,400 (160 × 15) that's probably sustaining her current weight.

You can reach that pound-a-week rate of loss through any combination of diet and exercise that eliminates or burns 500 calories a day

(3,500 calories a week)—as little as skipping a small bag of chips (3–3.5 ounces) each day. That, and a little patience, is what I'd recommend, both for ease of putting it into practice and the likelihood that the loss will be permanent.

You can step up the pace, however, if you so desire: Deleting 750 calories a day (one fast food taco salad, say, or one large milk shake) and adding a 250-calorie exercise burn daily (a 20-minute swim or run, 30 minutes of tennis or weightlifting or a 45-minute brisk walk) adds up to 2 pounds a week lost, close to the maximum safe rate for weight loss without losing muscle mass.

As you are setting your goals, be sure not to go below 12 times your *current* weight for daily calories. Our 160-pound woman should, by this reckoning, cut down to no fewer than 1,920 calories a day (160 × 12). Since she's probably sustaining 160 pounds on 2,400 calories a day, that's a difference of roughly the 500 calories a day we've been talking about, so at the 1,920-level, she would steadily reduce by about a pound a week, eventually stabilizing at about 128 pounds (128 × 15 = 1,920). On The Diet Code, weight loss counts only if it is

---

A CALORIE BY ANY OTHER NAME

If you're traveling in Europe and you want to find out how many calories a product contains, check the nutritional label for "energy." What a difference this one translation makes! Americans worry about how many calories a food has (and how fat we'll get from it), while Europeans are thinking simply about how much energy they'll get from that same food. It's all the same number, but here it has a negative connotation, and there it's a positive thing. It's just one hallmark of a food culture on much more of an even keel than our own. Whatever the word we use, the meaning we invest it with is up to us. I'm following Europe's lead and eating for energy.

truly fat loss (not water or muscle loss!) and only if it is undertaken in the service of good health. Weight loss that compromises your health is pointless, or worse.

No matter what your current or goal weight is, you don't want to go below 1,500 calories a day. After all, that's only enough to sustain a moderately active 100-pound person and will starve and/or malnourish any body much bigger than that (which is to say, just about everyone over 4 feet, 6 inches if kept up over any significant period of time). Chapter 9 lays out a menu plan pared back to this minimal level for those who want to drop weight as quickly as safely possible (definitely not the *easiest* way to do it), but even then it should be undertaken only for about a month at a time so you don't run into dehydration or catabolism of body tissue other than fat. I think you'll begin to see the problem with the myriad diets out there that, whatever their premise, tend to converge on one thing: diet plans of about 1,400–1,500 calories a day. You will lose weight initially, but you'll lose your health as well. And it will be difficult, and the weight is destined to return. Why mess with that? Here's one of the main advantages of The Diet Code: you lose weight by eating *more!*

Why should you shed pounds at The Diet Code pace when there are diets promising loss of a pound a *day*? Do the math. A 160-pound person would *have to stop eating altogether,* and even that would cut out only 2,400 of the necessary 3,500 calories each day. So even without food, they'd still need to burn over 1,000 calories daily—the equivalent of about two hours in the gym!

Balancing the Five Food Groups

Now, how are you going to take in however many calories you've decided is your target? Begin by choosing wisely from amongst the five food groups. To fill out your three main meals and three minimeals, you'll be making up to 15 choices from the five food groups. As a Journeyman, your choices should take best advantage of the most nutrient-dense foods of all (even within the Fundamental Foods grouping of highly nutritious foods). Include two servings every day of grains (G), two of lean protein (LP), two of starchy protein (SP), three of fatty protein (FP) and five of vegetables and fruits (VF) in any appealing combination at any given meal (while usually avoiding grain/starchy protein combinations that double up on rich carbohydrate sources, except for grains with dairy or beans). That's 14 selections all together, giving you another to play with, choosing again from whichever of the above you want.

Make variety a priority. Mix and match your favorite Fundamental Foods and explore new ones. Try different preparations. It keeps things interesting and ensures you're getting the widest range of nutrients.

On the other hand, keep it simple. Remember that you do not have to represent every food group at every meal. Nor does any group need more than one representative. Have a salad or a vegetable dish, but a healthy, balanced meal does not require both. Nor does it require grains *and* meat *and* vegetables to be complete. This less-is-more approach brings two benefits. One is easier meal planning, preparation and cleanup. Fewer ingredients to buy, fewer recipes to juggle, fewer dishes to wash. And two is that you'll want to eat less at any given meal. Studies show that even when they are already full, people will eat more when offered a new food that hasn't previously appeared at that meal—even when they turn down more of the same. The novelty appeals to us, and there's nothing wrong with that on its face, but we may as well use the knowledge to help us.

Realistically, you'll wind up with a week or so's worth of dishes you'll keep in regular rotation. As long as you are eating what you like and switching among a reasonable number of things, you won't get tired of anything, even if it hits your table once a week. The repetition of established favorites just plain makes life easier, using familiar dishes you know are nutritious and that everyone in your family will eat. Headliners will shift over time, no doubt, as some standards fall out of regular service and some newcomers seek center stage, so you'll keep or maintain variety that way!

Measuring Up to the Golden Ratio

As a Journeyman, you draw straight from the Fibonacci sequence (1, 1, 2, 3, 5, 8, 13 . . .) to create the Golden Ratio right there on your plate, nourishing yourself with a precise balance of Fundamental Foods from the five major food groups. This is a stricter approach and requires sizing food portions with a scale or sometimes a measuring cup. While this may seem demanding at first, it really takes only a few extra seconds—a worthy investment in the interest of reaching (and *staying at*) your ideal weight. Anyway, the point is as much to get a feel for the appropriate serving size as it is to get an exact portion on your plate. With regular practice, you'll soon know by instinct how much to serve yourself.

A kitchen scale is an indispensable Diet Code tool, especially for the Journeyman phase. If you've never used one before, let me assure you it is more convenient and efficient that you might realize. It's a far more accurate way to know exactly what you're eating—and therefore to create the Golden Ratio more precisely, and it's faster than measuring cups and spoons, too. Only with a scale will you be able to hit the Golden Ratio exactly. Throughout I've translated ounces into cups or tablespoons, trying to give you a feel for how much food I'm talking about in terms I'm sure are most familiar to most people. But as soon as you try it, you'll discover for yourself the problems with specifying whether 5 ounces of cantaloupe is ¾ cup or 1 cup. How big are your chunks, for one thing? Are you dicing it and mushing as much as possible into 1 cup? Or are your cubes so big only a few fit in, resting on each other with lots of air space filling the cup? There's a reason why nutritional reference information is given by weight. (Bakers deal only with weight. Flour can vary by 1 ounce per cup—that's a discrepancy of 25%!) If you, too, want accuracy, you, too, need to work with weight, not the far less consistent volume.

It requires something of a mental shift to think in terms of ounces instead of cups, but that is precisely the point. Once your default mode is weight, you'll be a much better Diet Code estimator. Learning to use the scale well is actually the best way to reach the point at which you no longer need to rely on it (though even I still throw things on the scale from time to time to check myself and to keep in practice).

You can get a mechanical 2- to 5-pound scale in any store that sells kitchenware. Most have a "tare" feature—check to make sure the one you select does—that automatically accounts for the weight of the container you are measuring anything in so you don't have to. Get one with a removable bowl for easy washing or, for flat-style scales, simply use your own light plastic container on top. It won't have to set you back any more than 30 to 40 dollars.

The chart below gives you a quick reference to general serving sizes and calorie counts for the most frequently used Fundamental Foods. Following that, I'll give you individual listings for specific Fundamental Foods you can use to get really precise. Through it all, see how the fingerprints of the Fibonacci sequence are all over this thing. When portioning out your food, you should aim for:

> 1–2 ounces FP (fatty protein): cheese, nuts, seeds, nut butter, olives, avocados
>
> 2–3 ounces G (grains): whole grain bread, pasta, cereal, whole grains
>
> 3–5 ounces LP (lean protein): fish, poultry, meat, tempeh, eggs, cottage cheese
>
> 5–8 ounces VF (vegetables and fruits): greens, tomatoes, peppers
>
> 8–13 ounces SP (starchy protein): potatoes, beans, peas, corn, yogurt

Just for fun, watch how the Fibonacci numbers (1, 2, 3, 5, 8 . . .) work if you measure these same servings another way: ⅛–⅕ pound of grain, ⅕–⅓ pound of meat, and ⅓–½ pound of vegetables!

Now for the central chart. You may recognize this from the Apprentice section, but this time, calorie counts have been added. The values

JOURNEYMAN
DIET CODE SERVING SIZES AND
CALORIES PER SERVING

Food Group	Serving Size	Calories
FP: *Fatty Protein*		
olives	1 oz (8–10 olives)	45
cheese	1 oz	110
nuts, seeds, nut butter	1 oz (2 tbsp nut butter, ¼ c whole nuts)	180
avocado	2 oz (¼ fruit)	80
ricotta	2 oz (¼ c)	110
G: *Grains*		
pasta, crackers, whole grains, bread, cereal, rice, polenta	2 oz (⅓ c) dry; 4–8 oz (⅔–1 c) cooked, depending on the grain or the noodle	200
Bavarian-style bread	2 oz (1 ⅜-inch-wide, 4-inch-square slice)	135
LP: *Lean Protein*		
cottage cheese, flaky white fish	3 oz (⅓ c)	90
tuna, chicken	3 oz (⅓ c)	140
eggs	2 (large)	140
tempeh	3 oz	140
steak	3 oz	225
VF: *Vegetables and Fruits*		
most vegetables, with 1 tsp olive oil	5 oz (1½ c)	100
winter squash, with 1 tsp olive oil	5 oz (1 c)	130
most fresh fruit	5 oz fresh (1 c)	85
most dried fruit	1½ oz dried (¼ c)	120
SP: *Starchy Protein*		
yogurt	8 oz (1 c)	130
potato (white)	8 oz (1 c)	185
beans	8 oz (1 c)	230

here have been rounded off, but accuracy remains high. The caveats from the Apprentice section about the inevitable range of values within each food group—the difference in the amount of food between 1.5 cups of spinach salad and 1.5 cups of cooked spinach, for example, or the difference in calorie density between carrots and lettuce grouped together under "vegetables"—still apply. (As a Journeyman, you can eliminate much of the variance by *weighing* your food [see "Measuring Up to the Golden Ratio" on p. 153] rather than scooping it out with measuring cups and spoons.) You'd have a whole book unto itself if you listed the specifics for every single food, but for those of you who would like more details still, you can find a wider variety of specific foods listed in appendix A, with carb, protein and fat content as well as serving sizes and calories.

Putting It Together

To get ready to assemble meals with the right calorie and macronutrient content for you, first determine how many calories you want to take in per meal. That depends, of course, or your total calorie target. Generally speaking, aim for between 400 and 700 calories for each main meal and between 100 and 400 calories per minimeal, finding your place within that range according to your daily total.

Of course, some days you might be lower on main meals and higher on minimeals, or vice versa, and as long as you stay within your total, that's fine. If for one snack you just have a piece of fruit, you'll have more calories to "spend" on another meal or snack that day. With you more in control of the energy your body is getting from what you eat, you can adjust the program in any number of ways without interfering with your weight loss or maintenance. That includes tipping the balance of the Golden Ratio on any given day (heavy on the carbs one day, say, or skimping on the fat) and compensating in a general way on another (minimizing carbs, to continue our examples, or getting extra fat). You can also go vegan on The Diet Code, or raise children on it, or fuel an athletic career on it. In the

Journeyman phase, you are in control of how the program flexes, as you create your own menus. Of course, you can also consult chapter 9 for plenty of Journeyman meal and menu ideas as well as chapter 10 for recipes and serving suggestions.

To give you just one example of how this all works, check out a day in the life of a 160-pound baker. My body uses 2,400 calories each day (160 × 15), so a typical slate of meals for me might look like what's on the next page. On this particular day, I got the recommended spread of selections from among the food groups (two grains, two lean proteins, two starchy proteins, three fatty proteins and five vegetables and fruits), filling in the remaining choice with an additional grain. You'll find much more along these lines in chapter 9.

Is This Golden?

Checking prepared or packaged foods with nutritional information on their labels for how they fit into The Diet Code is simple. The table on p. 159 shows the Golden Ratio of macronutrients (carbs, protein, fat) at several specific calorie levels, so you can gauge how any given food or dish measures up. Allowing wiggle room of about 10% is appropriate. A 200-calorie snack, perfect at 25 grams of carbs, 10 grams of protein and 6 grams of fat, would still be a good choice at 28 grams of carbs, 9 grams of protein and 5.5 grams of fat. Or, say you picked up a sports bar at the health food store and want to know if it would work as a Golden Ratio snack. Match up its calorie count to its carb, protein and fat gram content to see. And if it doesn't, this table could guide you in finding the right profile for a complementary food you could have with that energy bar to strike a balance. (This table appears again in appendix A, where it can be used, along with the more detailed listing of specific foods and their nutritional content included there, to analyze specific meals or food combinations for Journeyman who *really* want to roll their sleeves up and start working with the numbers.)

Here's how The Diet Code Macronutrient Profiles chart works:

MEAL	TOTAL CALORIES
Breakfast G-VF-SP	
Oatmeal (2 oz dry, 1 c cooked)	
Prunes (1½ oz, ¼ c)	
Yogurt (8 oz)	450
Snack G-FP	
Whole meal bread (2 oz)	
(1 ⅜-inch-wide 4-inch-square slice)	
Peanut butter (1 oz, 1 tbsp)	390
Lunch LP-VF-SP	
Tuna (3 oz), tomato (5 oz),	
bean (8 oz) and parsley salad (2 c)	410
Snack FP-VF	
Walnuts (1 oz, ¼ c)	
Apple (5 oz, 1 medium)	290
Dinner G-LP-VF	
Pasta (2 oz dry, 1 c cooked)	
Chicken (3 oz)	
Broccolini (5 oz)	
Beer (12 oz)	650
Dessert (snack) FP-VF	
Vento d'estate cheese (1 oz)	
Pear (5 oz, 1 medium)	210
	TOTAL: 2,400

You are aiming for 52% of your calories from carbs, 20% from protein and 28% from fat. As you might recall from chapter 2, there are 4 calories in 1 gram of carbohydrate, 4 calories in 1 gram of protein and 9 calories in 1 gram of fat. So if you are having a 100-calorie snack, for example, to make it in Golden Proportion, you'd want it to have 13 grams of carbohydrate: 52% of 100 calories is 52 calories. Fifty-two calories divided by 4 (calories per gram) gives you 13 grams of carbs. It works the same way for protein and fat: 20% of 100 calories is 20 calories; 20 calories divided by 4 (calories per gram) is 5 grams of protein. And 28% of 100 calories is 28 calories, divided by 9 (calories per gram) of fat, for a total of 3.1111. . . or 3 grams. Your Golden 100-calorie snack would have 13 grams of carbs, 5 grams of protein and 3 grams of fat, as the chart below summarizes for you. To save you the computations, I've done the math for serving sizes up to 700 calories.

DIET CODE MACRONUTRIENT PROFILES

Calories	Carbohydrates (in grams)	Protein (in grams)	Fat (in grams)
100	13	5	3
200	25	10	6
300	38	15	9
400	51	19	12
500	64	24	15
600	76	29	18
700	89	34	21

WINE AND BEER

The Diet Code easily accommodates a beer or a glass of wine with dinner, daily if you so choose. Just remember to include the calories in your calculations—replacing some other serving of grain (G) or starchy protein (SP). A 12-ounce bottle of beer has 150 calories, and the standard 5-ounce glass of wine has 106 calories.

ON THE SEVENTH DAY, REST

The Journeyman needs a regular break at least as much as the Apprentice does, so here again, take every seventh day off and eat whatever you want. You might turn it into a feast day or a fast day or anywhere in between as you grow more in tune with your body and its needs.

Don't be surprised, though, if you find the pull of your old habits waning. Your seventh-day menus might start to look much like those of the rest of the week, as what you really want to eat and what is good for you to eat come into alignment. Besides losing weight and looking great, you *feel* good on The Diet Code, and what you used to crave you may no longer find so appealing if it saps your energy or otherwise brings you down from that Diet Code high.

My three teenagers provide an excellent example of this. At home, they eat The Diet Code meals I cook, but when we're out, I always offer them whatever they want—cookies, candy, soda, ice cream. Yet, nine times out of ten they decline. They'll even push away some of their restaurant meals, saying it's "too much" pasta or "too much" meat. If you don't deny yourself, eventually you will find you are omitting many less than healthful things *without* feeling deprived. And still, you know there will always be room for that hot dog with the works when that's what you really want.

Moving On

You can expect to spend six months to a year in the Journeyman stage of The Diet Code. For at least a few months, you'll need to pay really close attention to calories, weighing and measuring out appropriate servings, checking Golden Ratio balances and so forth. By doing so, however, you will develop a feel for the amount of food that's good for you, and eventually you will be able to choose it without much conscious thought. You'll have an intuitive feel for what a meal looks like when it is proportioned properly. You're not thinking about food all the time; you simply know what and how much to pick, and you pick it. You'll invest less effort even as your results peak.

You won't worry about it if you have an ice cream cone once in a while; you'll be confident in knowing you have a system you can depend on. You'll know you can count on it, too, if you ever go off track with it, coming down with colds or putting on a few pounds. You can rewind to the conscious-effort phase for a refresher course if need be to get back into peak condition.

You'll have reached your ideal weight, and your weight will have stabilized right around there. You will be enjoying good health and abundant energy. Whatever goals you had for yourself in undertaking The Diet Code, you will have met them. What you hoped for, you will be experiencing. At this point, you will have reached Master territory.

It was up to you to decide when and if you wanted to move from Apprentice to Journeyman. But you don't decide to go on to the Master level. It just happens.

MASTER

The third phase of The Diet Code program is Master. With the return at the end of the journey, the hero is fully in touch with himself or herself—the hero has reached the master level. A master in any field of endeavor gauges a judgment on multiple and simultaneous inputs. When I was a carpenter, I could hear and smell the sharpness of a cutting tool beyond the coarser sense of touching the blade, and as a baker I can gauge the taste and quality of a loaf of bread just by looking at a photo of it. The synthesis of the senses, where one sense "fires" another, was given an official "diagnosis"—synesthesia—in the nineteenth century. Those who have it describe things like hearing the color blue or tasting shapes. Clinically, it's a rare phenomenon, and often quirky and subjective. But I believe anyone who completes a quest—anyone who reaches the return—can achieve a certain practical or useful integration of and mastery over the senses. It is, in fact, one of the hallmarks of the Master.

On The Diet Code, being a Master means you've reached the point at which eating this way no longer requires conscious effort. Your body, used to being fed whole foods, no longer has cravings for unhealthful foods. You've learned a lot, grown a lot, and now you've earned the right to relax your vigilance, knowing your knowledge will stand you in good stead no matter what. You'll be at the point where occasionally indulging in any food will not affect your overall weight or health. I throw something on the scale every once in a while now, just to check, but I don't keep up a hyper-vigilant state of measuring to the ounce. It used to be a useful tool, but it's one I no longer need to use on a regular basis. For many people, a Master-level appreciation can be achieved after about a year to a year and a half on the program.

The Master level isn't really a program at all. You reach this level once your body has fully adjusted to the natural foods and proportions it takes in on The Diet Code. You'll know intuitively when and what to eat, you won't have to measure or weigh anything and you won't be consciously counting calories. That's partly because you will have established good eating and exercise habits, partly because you'll recognize by sight what sustaining foods and proper portions and proportions are, and partly because you'll be in tune with how your body really feels. You'll be at a place where your weight has stabilized at a healthy level and, perhaps even more importantly, where you are happy, healthy and comfortable in and with your body. You'll be free of the "fear of food," knowing you are giving your body what it needs and having moved beyond unnecessary demonization of any one food or food group. Chapter 9 features a sample Master-level menu plan: mine.

The Master level is the understanding that you eat for health and happiness, not to specifically maintain your weight or for any other reason. You'll have fully rediscovered the sensual pleasures of eating and the essential vitality of really good food, and you'll eat with gusto and true appreciation. At this point, you'll set lifelong rhythms that are as natural as the flow of water. You'll be aware of your choices but not threatened or bound by them, and you'll be eating freely from inwardly established principles.

I keep my Master-level menu plan taped to my refrigerator, mainly so I don't miss a meal or forget to keep them varied. The portions I have down pat, but on busy days, I'm as prone as anyone to skipping a balanced meal. Even I could use a reminder from time to time to keep me at the top of my game. Right next to this Master diet guide, I post a Master workout guide. For me, it's referencing my martial arts practice. But I read it mainly as a workout for the head. I'll leave you with it now.

1. Improve incrementally. Improve. Incrementally. But improve.
2. Form comes first. Power and speed will follow.
3. Change up pace or speed of exercises to keep body improving. Incrementally.
4. Perform in five planes of movement. Up/down. Forward/backward. Side to side. Diagonal. Intentional.
5. Harder you go, harder you get. Incrementally. Intentionally.

The Seven-Course Lunch

A great living master, in my opinion, is Bill Coperthwaite. He was a woodworking mentor for me and a mathematical mentor, not to mention a huge fan of my bread. As such, he had a hand in guiding me into The Diet Code without ever knowing he was doing so. He doesn't officially follow The Diet Code—he's been eating his way long before the formal "plan" even existed—but his practices fit squarely within its guidelines. However, he pares it back to bare essentials. He customarily eats only one thing at any given meal so he can concentrate on and really enjoy it—usually a muesli of his own devising for breakfast, vegetables or fruit and cheese for lunch, and a steak for supper. So over the course of a day, he does create a Golden Ratio. In Bill's hands, it's as simple and uncomplicated as it could possibly be.

Bill is one of twin pillars of inspiration undergirding The Diet Code. The other is my grandfather. Both men truly appreciate their food, though in vastly different ways, and I aim for the same goal, always, for myself—via some middle way.

I began working with and for my grandfather when I was ten. Nono Gerry was the caretaker of a large estate, so his work involved every job in the world, it seemed to me: glazing windows, trimming rose bushes, fixing lawn mowers, building stone walls. But it was *work,* and he did it for 14 hours a day.

Except for half an hour for lunch. Watching my grandfather eat lunch was an experience. My cousin Rocco and I would wolf down our food and use the other 25 minutes to run races or get into mischief, chasing the chickens or something like that. But my grandfather took the full 30 minutes to eat his meal. Every day it was the same process. He'd open his domed aluminum lunch pail and pull out the seven-course Italian meal my grandmother had packed, laying everything out on a board. A Thermos of soup, a small dish of pasta with roasted peppers or olives or the like, a salad of some kind, two sandwiches (one with meat) and two desserts, fresh fruit and a baked dolce. I believe I witnessed most of the culinary wonders of Naples promenade across that plank through the four years I worked with Nono Gerry.

He ate slowly, reverently. Sometimes it seemed he was studying his food; always it seemed he was truly grateful for it. I can clearly remember how he'd gently open one particular folded wax paper packet each day as if it contained a sacred thing. And it did: a sandwich of peanut butter and banana on Italian bread, his favorite. He'd hold up this prize, turning it in the air, really looking at it, as if he were appraising a rare gem. He'd take a bite. And he'd say, every day, in his classic Italian-inflected English, "That's-a the best-a one!"

My grandfather always ate with such gusto, always with a truly *buon appetito.* He did good work, did it well, and never rushed anything, and he ate with the same intensity of dedication and pleasure. His skin was permanently tanned, and he always smelled like earth, inflected with a little garlic. And he was round, like a bowling ball. He and my grandmother had the same shape, padded by all that good food—it's the stature that's encoded in my DNA. Eating by The Diet Code, I've avoided that particular part of my inheritance. I didn't know it then, but the heart of The Diet Code was all there in that "best-a" sandwich: the combination of carbs, fat and protein—and the relishing of every bite.

The Diet Code is built on a foundation of ancient myth as well as ancient math. In other words, this artisan's approach is built to last. It may not be standing on the purely clinical studies bolstering doctor's diets, but those same clinical studies, like those promoting margarine, or linking high blood cholesterol to eggs, or blaming heart disease on beef, often seem to melt away like butter on hot toast. Some stand the test of time, of course, but in the service of fad diets, desperate and misappropriated science sends us down blind alleyways. And while there's a certain beauty in the scientific method, systems derived by that alone will always lack the intrinsic aesthetic appeal of something created by an inspired craftsman, adept both technically and artistically.

Part III

COOKING THE CODE

CHAPTER EIGHT

Taking Stock:
Pantry Tips and Cooking Techniques

Since most of us spend our lives doing ordinary tasks, the most important thing is to carry them out extraordinarily well.
—HENRY DAVID THOREAU

It's a little bit the fiddle but a whole lot more who holds the bow.
—WILBURN WILSON

Italians know how to turn the everyday into something special. They don't just make shoes; they make Perugia stiletto sandals. They don't just make cars; they make the Ferrari Maranello 575M. So it should be no surprise that when it comes to food, the Italians don't just make dinner.

That doesn't mean a meal has to be elaborate or particularly refined to be completely wonderful—and as nutritious as it is delicious. Distinction comes instead from selecting and preparing the best ingredients in the best way, which usually means with minimal interference. The next two chapters give you meal plans and recipes to launch you into The Diet Code, so this chapter will prepare you to undertake them with confidence.

With the advice given here on shopping and on stocking your pantry, you'll be ready to balance your macronutrients and Fundamental Foods in delicious meals even when you are short on time. The Diet Code requires no gourmet foods or rare ingredients; you can get most of the staples you need at your local supermarket or, better still, natural foods store, and here you'll learn how to always have just what you need on hand. A collection of preparation tips explains basic techniques for handling many of the Fundamental Foods that are aimed at maximizing efficiency and nutrition. You'll also get recommendations for the basic kitchen tools you'll need. For both food and equipment, having what you need—and only what you need—ready and waiting for you in the kitchen revolutionizes meal preparation into something not only manageable but also enjoyable.

Finally, the advice and instruction on essential classic Italian cooking techniques included in this chapter make following The Diet Code simple, allowing you to create wonderful meals in just minutes from readily available ingredients of the highest quality.

VINCENT AND PAUL

A scene from the movie *Vincent and Theo* (about the nineteenth-century impressionist painter Vincent van Gogh) delineates in a series of quick visuals just how wonderful a meal can be, given the right ingredients, tools and techniques—and just how wrong even a sincere effort can be without them.

Van Gogh is seen stirring a gray, glutinous muck of a stew when fellow painter Paul Gauguin comes home from the market bearing the makings of his own meal. Upon witnessing the pathetic efforts of his roommate, Gauguin throws his arm across the table to clear it of rusty implements and discolored potato peelings, then pours out his small cornucopia: baguette, soft cheese, ripe tomatoes and basil. He simply slices the tomatoes, dresses them and the basil leaves with olive oil and salt, and takes out a good bottle of wine. Dinner is ready.

You can pick your favorite painter. But when it comes to the kitchen, the purpose of this chapter is to put you directly in league with Gauguin. For this chapter, consider him a direct descendant of Leonardo—in the art of food, at least.

THE PANTRY

A fully stocked kitchen for The Diet Code will include regular supplies of the Fundamental Foods introduced in chapter 5, supplemented by a variety of artisanal and seasonal foods and personal favorites. Here I've pared it down for you, following a reductionist philosophy (honed over my years as a college student and bachelor), to the bare bones: just 20 items to keep on hand that are enough to meet basic nutritional needs *and* build dozens of delicious and blindingly quick Diet Code meal combinations. Stock your pantry with the minimum following convenient and common foods:

The Top 20

Whole meal bread or crackers

Oatmeal (or bulgur or rice)

Pasta

Canned beans

Onions

Carrots

Cabbage (or greens)

Fresh parsley

Crushed tomatoes

Apples

Lemons

Raisins (or prunes)

Canned tuna (or sardines)

Eggs

Peanut butter (or seed butter)

Yogurt (or kefir)

Olive oil

Grana (or other hard Italian cheese)

Sea salt

Cracked black pepper (or chile flakes)

Even if that was all you had, you'd have plenty of Diet Code meal options, including simple, classic combinations such as:

Apple and peanut butter

Oatmeal with yogurt with raisins

Bean stew

Pasta and tuna with lemon and parsley

Grilled apples and onions

172   COOKING THE CODE

Tuna stewed in tomato sauce with grated Grana
Pasta with cabbage and beans
Glazed carrots with raisins and lemon
Cabbage slaw with lemon and parsley and a hard-boiled egg

Condiments, Herbs and Spices

You'll be expanding your pantry, of course, filling it out with a fuller selection of Fundamental Foods (see the shopping list on p. 175 for further guidance). Once you do, you'll also want to have an array of condiments, herbs and spices on hand—the judicious application of which is what breathes life into many a meal. If you peeked into my cabinets on any given day, you'd probably find the following items:

Olive oil

Grapeseed oil

Sunflower oil

White balsamic vinegar

Aged red balsamic vinegar

Red wine vinegar

White rice vinegar

Orange marmalade

Thai fish sauce (anchovy base)

Thai sweet chili sauce

Thai hot chili sauce

Miso

Chicken/beef/ham bouillon

Nori seaweed flakes (with
    bonito and sesame seeds)

BBQ sauce

Honey

Turbinado semiraw sugar
    crystals

Rum

White wine

Sauerkraut

Kimchi

Salsa

Olives

Coarse sea salt

Black pepper (in pepper mill)

Fennel seed

Anise seed

Caraway seed

Saffron

Turmeric

Chile flakes

Juniper berries

Ground nutmeg

Ground coriander

Ground cinnamon	Fresh bay leaf
Ground clove	Fresh rosemary
Dried marjoram	Fresh basil
Dried (or fresh) oregano	Fresh sage
Dried (or fresh) mint	Fresh parsley
Dried (or fresh) thyme	

Now you've got plenty of options for spicing up any dish you're putting together, whether stirring orange marmalade into a marinade or dressing, sprinkling grilled veggies with aged balsamic or the nori flakes, spiking seared fish with rum or white wine, or topping eggs and beans with salsa. I like warm spices like ground cinnamon and nutmeg with winter squash; aromatics like caraway and fennel with cauliflower, cabbage and potatoes; saffron or turmeric when I need a little color and a mouthwatering bitter edge; Thai sweet chili sauce and a bay leaf on broiled white fish; fresh oregano leaf for grilled beef; sage on chicken or white beans; and, of course, basil with just about any form of tomato.

SHOPPING

As we learned from Gauguin and van Gogh, an excellent meal begins with smart shopping. To the degree you can, shop like an Italian— walking to the market daily gets you not only the freshest foods but also a bit of exercise. In addition, not having endless supplies of every food item imaginable on hand can reduce temptation. Sure, stock up on brown rice and crushed tomatoes and the like, but nothing good is going to come from having big bags of chips in the cupboard at all times or looking at half-gallons of ice cream every time you open the freezer. Buy junk food occasionally if you must—not as a matter of habit—and buy it in single-serving sizes. That way, you can eat 1.5 to 2 ounces of chips, for example, and be done. There's no danger of working your way to the bottom of a full-size bag.

Shop local and buy artisanal as much as possible, and choose organic whenever you can. At your local grocery store, focus on the shelves lining the outside walls—that's where the fresh, whole food is always located. The inner aisles harbor the more processed and preserved foods. The same goes for the health food store. Make forays to the interior for canned beans, dried pasta, tinned tuna and so on, but more should come from the produce, dairy, fish and bakery sections. I lived for many years as a homesteader with only a root cellar for refrigeration, and to this day the only things you'll find in my freezer are coffee beans and glasses icing for white wine or a frosty beer. If you prefer a fuller freezer, I'd advise stocking it with your own preportioned Diet Code dishes. Commercially prepared frozen goods are, in the main, too refined and processed. But Diet Code meals are so quick to make that I don't think you'll find it any advantage to start with frozen ingredients. That just means adding on defrosting time! Having some plain veggies in the freezer might be useful for times when fresh is not an option.

Get in the habit of reading labels, checking for recognizable natural ingredients. Note—and obey!—the recommended serving sizes and servings per container; most times, they match Diet Code proportions.

You'll find that familiarity with Diet Code proportions simplifies shopping. You'll *know* a pound of meat can feed four and that a pound of rice makes two meals for four. How much you need to buy will always be clear, streamlining shopping decisions, not to mention cutting down on food waste. The conservative serving sizes also allow you to afford higher quality, handmade and organic selections. Instead of a 12-ounce steak flaccid from commercial feed and growth hormones, you can afford a 4-ounce cut of the best grass-fed beef. Fueling the demand for the healthiest product—both for humans and for the planet—can be your personal contribution to a Renaissance of real food.

The Shopping List

To speed up shopping, make a master list for the kitchen and hone it by grouping the items by location headings or aisle numbers. My own list expands around the top 20 previously listed and includes both general ("other fruit") and specific ("oranges") items to accommodate what's seasonal or on special at the store, as well as what I already have in mind to cook that week or know I am out of. Add a separate section for what you need to pick up at specialty shops, like the fish market, wine store or butcher. For my family of four, this

MY GROCERY SHOPPING LIST		

Vegetables
Cabbage
Carrot
Onion
Garlic
Pepper
Tempeh
Greens
Other
	Dairy
	Eggs
	Yogurt
	Cottage cheese
	Ricotta cheese
	Piave or Grana
	   (my favorite Italian
	   hard cheeses)
	Other
		Oils
		Olive
		Sunflower
		Grapeseed
		Other

Fruit
Apple
Banana
Oranges
Lemon/lime
Other
	Canned
	Crushed tomatoes
	Butter/cannellini
	   beans
	Red kidney/adzuki
	   beans
	Black beans
	Chickpeas
	Tuna
	Sardines/herring
	Lentils (dry)
	Other
		Nuts/Dried Fruit
		Peanut butter
		Sunflower seed
		   butter
		Hemp butter
		Flaxseed
		Nut mixes
		Raisins
		Prunes/figs
		Other

Deli
Fish
Smoked fish
Bacon
Chicken sausage
Other
	Grains
	Brown rice
	Bulgur
	Oatmeal
	Bread
	Other
		Pasta
		Penne
		Quinoa elbows
		   or rotelle
		Rice noodles
		Spelt soba
		Kamut gemelli
		   or fusilli
		Other

technique reduces shopping to about an hour a week because I thread my way through the stores rehearsed and with purpose.

Best Brands

Here are some specific brands and types to look for, all of which I buy in my local health food store and supermarket. In case what you want is not on the shelf, I've supplied some Internet and mail-order sources, many of which provide a wealth of information on a wide variety of natural whole food products.

Breads
Sprouted Grain Bread
Ezekiel 4:9: www.food-for-life.com

Westphalian/Bavarian-Style Bread
Schnitzer organic spelt (German import): Anke Kruse Organics,
    Inc., www.ankekruseorganics.ca
Mestemacher (German import)
Hümmlinger (German import): 800-818-7729
Genuine Bavarian (German import)

Bouillon
Harvest Sun Organic Free-Range Chicken Cubes (German
    import): Anke Kruse Organics, Inc.,
    www.ankekruseorganics.ca
Seitenbacher Instant Broth (vegan German import)
Organic Gourmet Wild Mushroom Concentrate (German
    import): www.organic-gourmet.com

Nuts and Seeds
Hemp seed, meal and butter: www.manitobaharvest.com,
    www.livingharvest.com, www.rejuvenative.com

Seed and nut butters: Grain & Salt Society,
www.celtic-seasalt.com (an extensive Web site, and obviously a
good source of natural sea salt as well)

Tomatoes
Pomi by Parmalat (aseptic pack) (Italian import)
Mutti Chopped Tomatoes (aseptic pack) (use 1½ of the
standard-size 18-ounce cartons in recipes calling for a
28-ounce package)

Specialty Vegetables and Greens
Four Seasons Farm, Barbara Damrosch and Eliot Coleman,
Cape Rosier, Maine: www.fourseasonfarm.com

Dairy
Woodstock Water Buffalo yogurt and fresh mozzarella: Star Hill
Dairy, www.woodstockwaterbuffalo.com
Redwood Hill Farm goat milk yogurt: www.redwoodhill.com
Kefir: www.heliosnutrition.com
Yogurt: Seven Stars Farm, 610-935-1949

Pasta and Grains
Fusco bronze die imported Italian pasta
Castellana Rustic Italian imported pasta
Rustichella d'Abruzzo pasta (Italian import):
www.manicaretti.com
Giuseppe Cocco/Fara San Martino pasta (Italian import)
Barilla Plus Multigrain pasta
Organic pasta from Italy: www.bionaturae.com
Ezekiel 4:9 brand sprouted multigrain pasta
Quinoa pasta: Quinoa Corporation Ancient Harvest:
www.quinoa.net
Kamut-, spelt- and quinoa-blend pastas: www.edenfoods.com
Farro (semipearled Umbrian spelt): www.rolandfood.com

Spelt/kamut/millet/buckwheat flours and grain flakes:
   www.arrowheadmills.com
Organic grains and flours: www.lundberg.com

Granola
Grandy Oats: www.grandyoats.com

Food Bars
For starters, you should only consider eating all-natural energy bars
with pure ingredients, not one loaded up with more chemicals than
real food. Even then, many (if not most) of them are so loaded with
carbs that they are really only appropriate for when you're getting a
heavy workout of some kind and need the extra. Then, too, you want
to make sure the macronutrients are in reasonable balance; the key
here is to start with one with sufficient protein. I like to look for
10 grams of protein per bar. Then, I try to get as close to Diet Code
proportions as I can—ideally, 6 grams of fat and 26 grams of carbs to
go with those 10 grams of protein—in about 200 calories. The first
two bars listed below fit this profile reasonably well. The others
aren't as close but are still nutritious and made from whole foods. You
may want to consider eating them with a little something on the side
to complete the balance.

Greens+ Natural Energy Bar: www.greensplus.com
Zoe's Flax and Soy Bar: www.zoefoods.com
Organic Food Bar (vegan): www.organicfoodbar.com
Gertrude & Bronner's Magic Alpsnack bars: www.alpsnack.com
Kelp Krunch Sesame Bar: Maine Coast Sea Vegetable, Inc.,
   www.seaveg.com
Govindas Hempbar: 800-900-0108

Bacon/Pork Sausage
North Country Smokehouse: www.ncsmokehouse.com
Sunset Acres Farm and Dairy: www.sunsetacresfarm.com, 207-
   326-4741 (also a great source for eggs and goat cheese)

Preparation Tips: Shortcuts to Selecting and Preparing Fundamental Foods

Veggies

When it comes to shopping for vegetables at a supermarket (as opposed to a farmers' market), choosing the best varieties can be key. Opt for organic whenever you can, of course, but that's not the end of the story. Though the real thing (from local small farms) will always be best, commercial peppers are good, as are kale and collard greens, leeks, onions and garlic. Check out filet beans (a.k.a. French beans or haricot verts) rather than the fibrous, watery green beans usually sold right beside them. They are much tastier, sweeter and even a little meaty, and they don't have the big, dull seeds of their more familiar cousin.

It's no surprise to me that so many people hate broccoli, though: The stuff available in the supermarket tastes pretty terrible, sulfurous and tough. (Organic, when you can find it, is worlds better, especially if it has slimmer stalks.) If you like it, have at it. But for a happy and tastier alternative, give broccolini a try. This ancient version, newly rediscovered and brought back to the mass market, has thinner, more tender stems and lots of clean, slightly peppery flavor. Even your kids may love it.

Greens

Wash and slice greens ahead of time and store them in the fridge. To reduce your time spent in the kitchen at dinnertime as well as to ensure ideal Diet Code serving sizes, stuff 5- to 6-ounce portions into individual plastic bags. These single servings can be deliciously braised in a skillet or even a microwave with olive oil, garlic and a bit of smoked bacon in a few minutes (see recipe on p. 285) to make an impromptu fresh side dish for a quick can of chili, tuna salad or precooked sausage. Wouldn't you rather grab a moment with a Frisbee while the sun's out than cook? (Or is that an idea you have to be a New Englander to truly appreciate?)

Beans

Though admittedly none tastes as good as dry beans well soaked and slow simmered, you should stock a few cans of your favorite varieties of precooked beans to put a meal in reach in minutes.

You could save yourself a bit of cleanup in the bargain: In Leonardo's Tuscany, beans were cooked by putting them in a jar or flask filled with water set near the fire to bake slowly. Sometimes the expansion was too much for the flask (or *fiasco*)—hence our use of the word *fiasco* to connote a failure or a mess.

Preparing beans still requires careful attention so you can avoid a similar fate, as anyone who's ever inexpertly handled a pressure cooker for the task knows. Beans that aren't well cooked cause digestive trouble, too (also of an explosive nature!), so be sure to soak them long enough and to cook them thoroughly.

Tomatoes

Tomatoes absolutely must be of high quality or they are simply not worth eating. If you can't get fresh, farm-grown tomatoes in season, you're better off with crushed or chopped tomatoes or tomato sauce in aseptic paper cartons than you are with the mealy and tasteless hothouse atrocities supermarkets try to pass off. I did a taste test with my customers one day, making some pizza with packaged crushed tomatoes and some with the most reasonable fresh tomatoes to be had from the grocery store, and my eager volunteers chose the former every time. The aseptic packaging preserves the freshest taste and is free of the metallic overtones that are often present in tomatoes packed in cans. You can't go wrong looking for tomatoes imported from Italy.

Fruit

Berries last no more than a few days, and seasonal fruits at the peak of ripeness don't stick around either. But making frequent trips to the market to keep a supply on hand is definitely worth it. Apples, oranges and bananas are the sturdiest fruits to keep continually on hand. Fruit juice may seem like a good solution, but without the fiber you get from whole fruit, the juice is concentrated in sweetness and in calories, and therefore you should drink it infrequently as a treat.

Bread

The most nutritious breads are the slow-baked sourdough whole meal types originating in the geographic belt from northern Italy to Romania. These Bavarian- and Westphalian-style breads (similar to my *mattone*) can be found in health food stores and large supermarkets in thinly sliced 1-pound squarish loaves, in vacuum packed or foil wrapped packets. Many varieties are wheat free and even flourless, containing just crushed whole grains. Ezekiel 4:9 brand and other sprouted grain breads are chewy and satisfying and also merit a place at the top of the list for good nutrition. Look for both sandwich loaves and pita rounds. And, of course, seek out your local bakery specializing in handcrafted sourdough loaves. Most often, you should choose the whole grain varieties there, with a well-made country sourdough baguette or peasant bread thrown in every now and then. Artisanal sourdough white bread is healthier than any store brand "multigrain" or "wheat" breads, which are only marginally different from Wonder™ bread.

To help you gauge how much bread to buy, keep in mind that a 1-pound loaf will generally get four people through two meals. On The Diet Code, each person in your household will probably be eating 4 to 6 ounces (¼–⅓ pound) of bread daily (two servings a day).

When it comes to making your own bread, the most important thing to remember is that you *must* weigh your flour—there's too much discrepancy from cup to cup if you just scoop it. So if my baking recipes look a little funny, that's why. It's also the reason so many baking recipes fail you—flour measured in cups will never provide consistent results. Liquid and granular things (like milk and sugar) can be measured with measuring cups rather than weighed because the amount you get is constant each time you fill a cup.

Poultry and Meat

Selecting meat carefully is key. Whenever you can find and afford it, choose vegetarian/grass-fed, free-range, organic and antibiotic-free chicken, turkey, lamb and beef. You will taste the difference between them and factory-produced supermarket meats. And you'll find that you eat less of the higher quality stuff because you'll be more readily satisfied. So if you think about price per meal rather than price per pound, the good stuff isn't really more expensive. If you're still feeling like you can't afford it, consider the long-term costs of health complications, environmental degradation and agricultural unsustainability that you're buying into along with your mass-market meat. Then relax and enjoy an all-natural 3- to 4-ounce rib eye rather than a huge slab of cheap steak.

My favorite meat is turkey, which I often buy in cutlets and tenderloins (great for satay-style grilling) as well as the usual legs, wings, thighs and breast parts. And I always keep a pack of precooked organic chicken sausage on hand for use in a range of 5- to 15-minute meals (see recipes).

Cheese

The Europeans as a whole have the edge when it comes to making cheeses, but outstanding cheeses are now being produced in small batches by artisans in New Hampshire, Maine, Vermont, New York and across the country.

If you are inclined toward mainstream cheeses like cheddar, Swiss or Monterey jack, precut the blocks into 1-ounce portions. Simply divide the typical half-pound (8-ounce) bar into eight pieces, so the perfect size is ready and waiting when you need a companion for bread, crackers or fresh fruit.

Pasta

I generally use dried pasta for simplicity of acquisition, storage and cooking. Anything you can find imported from Abruzzi—the reigning region for pasta-making, singled out because of the way wheat is grown there—is going to be worthwhile. Look for handmade pastas, which are air dried (not flash dried, which means baked in an oven. This oxidizes out flavors as well as nutrients). Artisans use bronze dies to cut and shape their pasta. This method dates back to Roman times and texturizes the surface of the pasta so it holds sauce better.

To cook any pasta, bring salted water to a boil in a stockpot, and then add the noodles. Quinoa and rice pastas will be ready 4 to 6 minutes after hitting the water, while wheat pastas (kamut, spelt and buckwheat as well as the classic durum semolina) need 6 to 10 minutes. Test for doneness after the shortest suggested cooking time has elapsed so you can be sure to get the pasta off the heat when it is done *al dente*. That provides a particularly satisfying texture and is definitely the Italian way of doing things. But even more important for The Diet Code is the fact that this allows for a slower breakdown of starches as you digest the pasta, lowering its glycemic index so you can eat it without negatively impacting your blood sugar levels or your waistline.

Another way to lower the glycemic index of pasta is with a squeeze of lemon juice or any citrus. Think pasta with seafood and lemon, pasta with zucchini and lemon, and so on. It's this trick that makes tabouli (bulgur with parsley, tomatoes, mint and lemon) low in glycemic impact and part of the formula for Alpine Baked Porridge Muffins (see recipe on p. 269).

Olive Oil

Olive oil stays fresh for about a year and will be reasonably good for another year after that, but thereafter the flavor and aroma will start to decline, along with its health benefits. Now, a bottle of good olive oil would never last that long in my house, but you also have to remember that any oil has been stored in the bottle for a while before it ever reaches your kitchen. Dark bottles are best, as light can denature the oil. For the same reason, you should store whatever bottle you have in a dark cabinet. Heat breaks down olive oil as well, so don't waste your finest on sautéing or grilling. Use inexpensive ones when you are cooking, and drizzle the ones with the desired flavor on top when you're done.

Nuts and Seeds

Prewrap ¼-cup (1½-ounce) servings of nut mix in twists of waxed paper so you'll always have the right serving size ready to go.

Whole Grains

Cooking whole grains is generally very simple. Here's a guide to get you started.

EASY COOKING GUIDE			
GRAIN	**MEASURE PER SERVING**	**WATER PER SERVING**	**TO COOK**
Rolled oats	⅔ c (2 oz)	1 c	Microwave 1 minute.
Couscous, kasha (toasted buckwheat)	⅓ c (2 oz)	⅔ c	Bring water to boil. Pour in grains. Stir once. Remove from heat and cover. Let stand for 15 minutes.
Quinoa, bulgur, white rice	⅓ c (2 oz)	¾ c	Bring grain and water to a boil over medium-high heat. Reduce heat to medium and cover. Cook 15 minutes. Remove from heat and let stand for 15 minutes more.
Amaranth	⅓ c (2 oz)	⅔–¾ c	As above, but cook 20–25 minutes.
Millet	¼ c (2 oz)	1¼ c	As above, but cook 30–35 minutes.
Brown and wild rice	⅓ c (2 oz)	1 c	As above, but cook 40 minutes.

KITCHEN EQUIPMENT

The foods stocking your pantry are like the body of the fiddle, and the utensils are like the bow, the tool that works it.

I have the same philosophy of simplicity about equipment in my kitchen as I do about food in my larder. Most guests are shocked at how few gadgets I use in the kitchen. Through three decades, I've pared the list to a capable set of less than 50 items to cover all the cooking in The Diet Code. If you're a big kitchenware collector, I won't knock your hobby. It's just that I like spending less time at the stove and the sink and more time at the table. As the Italian proverb states, *A tavolo non s'invecchia*—we do not age at the dinner table.

In the end, though, a 200-dollar sauté pan can't make you a good cook. In fact, too many items in your kitchen, no matter how fine or dear, will eventually impede rather than improve your cooking. I buy commercial-style pans at kitchenware shops in the 30- to 40-dollar range that I am quite pleased with, even as admittedly picky as I am about well-made tools. And I keep no more in my kitchen cabinets and drawers than I need to make everyday meals. So it's never a struggle to find the ladle in a jumbled drawer or an ordeal to wrestle the right pot out from under a pile of competitors or futile to try to find the matching lid.

A streamlined kitchen speeds cleaning as well as cooking. A professional chef, for example, can do almost everything with just a knife and tongs, meaning he or she spends less time looking for gadgets and washing up a sinkful of them. Simplifying the process allows you to focus your energy on the food, and that extra care translates into a better-tasting meal.

The following lists assume you have a basic kitchen setup with stove top, sink, refrigerator and oven. They are organized with the most important items first, in case you want to pare back further.

Utensils

10 Essentials:

- 12- to 16-inch light stainless hinged tongs (These are so handy that they can replace a whole drawer full of spoons and spatulas and other miscellany.)
- Pot holder/oven mitt (Because I'm a baker, I tend to do a lot of work that others might do on the stove top in the oven, so I like the new silicone mitts and slide-on handle insulators. They allow pans to be moved from stove top to oven safely. The silicone holders are very sanitary and don't collect oils, like the cloth versions do.)
- Hand-crank can opener (There is no need for a counter-hogging electric version of a tool you'll use only a few times a week.)
- Waiter's style corkscrew/bottle opener (Like the can opener, this tool rates high not because you'll use it every day but because you really can't do without it when you need it!)
- 6- to 8-inch fine stainless wire sieve (This is useful for straining liquids, broths and sauces and as a mini colander for draining a can of beans or tuna.)
- Soup ladle
- 14-inch light nylon pancake turner
- 12- to 14-inch bamboo or wooden spoon (This is good for many tasks you could also accomplish with the tongs, but you'll often appreciate the quiet of wood on metal rather than metal on metal.)
- Scissors (Anything you'll do with them in the kitchen could also be done with a knife, but for the average cook, scissors provide an advantage in both safety and convenience.)
- Pepper mill (There's nothing like the piquant sharpness of freshly ground pepper to coax out the most flavor; for the same reason, a salt mill is also an excellent, though not strictly necessary, addition.)

(Second) Best Bets:

You can do without these if pressed, but these nine sure are helpful:

- 10- to 14-inch rubber mixing spatula
- Whisk
- Skimming ladle: stainless mesh or copper wire basket (This is a big help in blanching vegetables and poaching fish or pasta like ravioli.)
- Plastic squeeze bottles for cooking oils (Keep one for fruity olive oil and one for light cooking oil, like sunflower and/or grapeseed, and enjoy the ability they give you to more carefully control the amount you use and the amount of mess you make—all using just one hand!)
- Disk-style potato masher (It is handy for many mashing jobs— I often use it for winter squash "puree" and bean spreads like hummus—that others might haul out the food processor for. Sometimes, doing it by hand is simply more efficient. Labor-saving devices are great, but only if they really do save you time.)
- Garlic press (Professional chefs mash cloves with the side of a blade and then mince them fine.)
- Bulb baster
- Gelato/ice cream scoop (You might only use it once a week, but it will save your dinner spoons from bending.)
- Electric hand or stand mixer

Knives

A sharp knife makes food look and taste fresher. That dexterous professional chef mentioned above accomplishes so much with little more than a knife by putting all its parts into action: cutting edge, heel, tip, spine, side and handle. In 30 years, I've never found a need for more than three knives at home:

- 7- to 8-inch chef's knife
- 3- to 4-inch paring knife
- 10- to 12-inch serrated bread knife

Cutting Tools

- Diamond hone (knife sharpener)
- Vegetable peeler
- Cheese grater (And use it! Don't bother with flavorless, pre-grated stuff.)
- Cheese shaver (because on grilled vegetables, like asparagus or zucchini, even freshly grated cheese doesn't cut it)
- Chopping block/cutting board for vegetables (sturdy wooden one measuring about 16 by 24 by 1¾ inches)
- Cutting board for meat—12- by 16-inch wood or nylon with perimeter blood groove (Use one side for cutting raw meat and the other for cutting cooked roasts. Reserve your larger chopping board for vegetable prep only.)
- 11-cup food processor (if you like; I don't have one at home myself because I find doing it by hand is almost always more efficient when you factor in cleaning and storing your equipment. I do use one in my café, mainly for making bean spread and chopping nuts.)

Measuring Tools

- 2-cup beaker measure
- 5-pound kitchen scale
- Timer
- Measuring spoons, light stainless steel (¼ tsp–1 tbsp)
- Light plastic or stainless measuring cups (¼–1 cup)
- Meat thermometer

Prep Bowls

- Two mixing bowls, light stainless steel, 10–14 inches
- Colander, 12-inch light stainless steel
- Salad spinner, good quality plunger style

Cooking Pans

- 12-inch nonstick ovenproof covered skillet
- 8- to 12-quart covered heavy-bottom stockpot of 18/10 stainless steel (not aluminum)
- 2½ quart heavy covered saucepan
- 10- to 12-inch square nonstick grill pan with deep (2-inch) sides (a type of ovenproof skillet, often square, with a rippled bottom that allows you to mimic the grilling process without the grill)
- 4-quart ovenproof enameled cast-iron covered casserole
- 5½- and 9-inch hard plastic microwavable containers with covers
- 12- by 16- by 3-inch nonstick roasting pan with rack
- Optional smaller 8-inch skillet for backup

Baking Pans

- 10-inch round or square removable-bottom cake pan
- 11- by 17-inch (or 12- by 16-inch) heavy aluminum or insulated-bottom cookie sheet/bake pan
- Parchment baking paper
- Vegetable oil spray
- "Texas-sized" muffin tin (and paper muffin cup liners)

GET COOKING

A simple yet wonderful meal like the one Gauguin assembled is what Italians call *alla cruda*—raw or, literally, done crudely. In the movie, it is the culinary art that shows van Gogh's kitchen disaster for what it was. Fathoms removed from the gruel van Gogh was laboring over, Gauguin's offering brought to the table a healthy pantry and appropriate technique—in this case just a slash and a splash.

Maximizing taste and nutrition, even from fresh ingredients, requires appropriate skills. Becoming a good cook is, like any craft, usually not innate but learned. I used to make frightfully bad dishes faulted mainly by the use of too little fat and too many herbs or seasonings. Sloppy knife work, bad cookware, mismatched techniques and trying to cook everything all at once—like a sodden stir-fry— are the other major impediments I (and possibly you) needed to overcome to turn out a decent meal. Even the best ingredients, if mishandled, make a far worse meal than average stuff masterfully brought to the plate. Aim, of course, to start with the best and treat it the best way.

The finest meals balance the raw with the rendered (those parts of a meal shaped by cooking, like Gauguin's loaf of bread). As soon as humans mastered fire, they started developing cooking techniques, first grilling over coals, and in short order smoking, plank grilling, spit roasting and baking. Heated stones dropped into water-filled hollowed logs; and bark, animal-hide or even sewn-leaf containers scalded and boiled foods for early man before fireproof pots. As earthenware and metalworking capabilities evolved, applications of fire and water interfaced into syntheses: steaming, stewing, blanching, sautéing, poaching, braising, reduction glazing.

By the fifteenth century, Leonardo's time, the Italians had already amassed and perfected a compendium of culinary techniques that remain to this day in need of no amendment. French cuisine, the world's most elaborate outside of authentic Chinese, was an Italian inheritance: After Caterina de Medici's marriage to the French king

Henry II in 1533, she forcibly installed a Tuscan kitchen staff of 40, leaving behind the barbaric cooking methods of the Gauls and giving wing to the new gastronomical flights of France and greater Europe. Unfortunately, court distinction persuaded Caterina to put on airs, and she cropped her native mangiafagioli, or bean-eating, trait, replacing it with unhealthy changes. In her wake, the regal palate grew to decadent extremes, the perfect example being Marie Antoinette's famous eighteenth-century insistence on white carbs ("Let them eat cake!") in the run-up to the French Revolution. We're still struggling with a royal disdain for vegetables and preference for refined carbs that came down to us.

The Fiddler

How you go about doing something makes all the difference in the outcome—like the contrast between the meals of Gauguin and van Gogh at table. My techniques are informed by a combination of classical Italian skills and more homely secrets I learned by watching my grandmother in the kitchen, offset by observing my own working parents endeavor to get a meal on the table at the end of the day.

At the point in her life when I knew her, Nona Louisa always cooked with a bounty of fresh foods, thanks to the gardens and chicken coops she tended so carefully. Fresh produce still reigns in my household as well as in my business, which I credit her with as much as I do my abilities with cooking Italian classics.

From my mom I first gleaned some shortcuts. Soup stock made from a roast chicken or turkey carcass is incomparable, no question, but at the end of a workday, using a (quality) bouillon cube instead makes a 15- to 20-minute meal possible. I've also learned to incorporate canned beans and a few commercial condiments, as described on p. 172.

But my mom's true forte is presentation—the arrangement of shape, texture and color. She's the ultimate hostess, and her spreads are revered. Years later as a homesteader weathering a Maine winter with only potatoes or bread and oil and spruce-needle tea on the table, I called on her method to make them look *really* good to eat.

My dad was a grill master: sausage and peppers, lobster or clams, garden vegetables and, of course, steak. Childhood summers featured pretty much one preparation, and to tell you the truth, I really couldn't have been happier about it. My living arrangements preclude the regular use of a charcoal-filled Weber—or any other outdoor cooking method. But Nona Louisa never cooked outdoors, either, yet her black-tinged "grilled" peppers and roast meats schooled me about the wonders of what can be done in this regard in an oven.

Cooking Techniques

A lack of culinary skill is a major setback to good eating, but Italian techniques are fortunately very simple to grasp. Here we'll review a dozen of the most common and useful Italian cooking techniques.

I'll start with the linchpin concept:

Insaporire, from the Latin word meaning tasty. It's more of an ultimate goal than a specific technique, a direction to coax flavor out of whatever you are preparing. Insaporire can be revealed in a proper dressing (lemon/oil/caper/anise), or a *soffrito* (frying bacon, garlic, minced herbs or vegetables in oil) to infuse a flavor base in a dish, or in singeing for char, or glazing fruit for carmelization, or simply recognizing peak ripeness, or plunging vegetables into cold water to arrest the cooking process and retain their texture. It's using everything you know and have access to in order to make that dish taste as good as it can be. All the other techniques below are done in the service of insaporire.

All cooking comes from two parents: desiccation or dry heat (baking, or *al forno*) and hydration or cooking wet (boiling, or *bollire*). From these twin roots, beginning with baking, spring:

Alla brace, to grill over coals (or broil). This sears the outside, sealing in the juices and keeping the food moist on the inside and especially tasty. Cooking on a grill also lets any excess fat melt off and caramelizes what remains for an additional richness of flavor. Both meat and vegetables—and sometimes even fruit—are good alla brace. If you don't have an outdoor grill (or outdoor grill *weather*), you can get the same results with a grill pan preheated in the top third of an oven that's as hot as you can make it, about 500 to 550 degrees Fahrenheit.

Salto is to sear or quickly brown or char the outer surface of a food, either on a flat surface over coals, in the oven or in a hot skillet over the stove top. This works much the same as grilling, though you don't get those great seared stripes. In addition, the food sits in any fat that melts off as it cooks, basting in flavor.

Saltere, or sauté, is essentially a milder searing process. Meat will self-baste; with vegetables, you add a little fat to get the same effect. Here again, browning or spotting the outside increases flavor.

On the wet side (boiling), we have:

Sobollire, a light boil or simmer, with tiny champagnelike bubbles gently breaking at the surface. (A full boil is so vigorous that it is rarely used in good cooking—the exception being for dry pasta—because it can break food and rob it of flavor.) Even a light boil releases flavor and nutrients into the cooking liquid, so this technique is used for soups or other dishes in which the food is going to be served in the cooking liquid. You might also use it for preparing whole root vegetables when their skins will keep the nutrients from leaking into the water. (If you need them cut up, do it *after* they are cooked.)

Affogato is the delicate simmer you may know as poaching. Using water or broth, this gently steaming pot is great for cooking delicate seafood, fish, vegetables and eggs you don't want to break up as they cook. Because you use a lower temperature than for sobollire, you'll lose fewer nutrients into the cooking liquid. Still, think about using this method to prepare dishes in which you're going to drink the broth.

Pippiare is using a light simmer for a long time to gently stew food. This is good for tougher foods that need some time to become tender, such as poultry or root vegetables, or for cooking dried beans. This can be done in the oven as well as on the stove top. Either way, you'll still want the broth to be integral to the finished dish so you don't toss out that flavor and nutrition with the cooking water. Think about how you make soup stock from carcasses (another great time to use pippiare). The whole point is to leach all the goodness out of the bones and into the broth.

Sbollentare is to scald, or heat up to just below a boil. This is the technique for thick, sensitive liquids like sugar syrups or cream- or cheese-enhanced dishes like chowders and pastry cream.

Ridurre is to reduce a liquid by simmering it. It thickens a liquid, concentrating and intensifying flavors, making it essential for creating sauces, gravies and excellent soup stock.

Brasato, or braising, is one of the most important yet often overlooked techniques. It is a hybrid of wet and dry, sort of a steam / sauté in which a small bit of liquid (often the water left on vegetables after rinsing) and/or fat (cooking oil) is added to a hot skillet. This is *the* technique for preparing most vegetables, particularly green vegetables, and makes the most brilliant and tasty greens. I never, ever steam vegetables. (I don't like them that way. Does anybody, really?) Brasato is the way to go. It's also good for cuts of meat that need help staying tender and moist.

Soffocato, or "choking," is a long, slow braise on top of the stove or in the oven, perfect for tough or inexpensive cuts of meat or game. This is what the Italians are doing when they throw a pot on the back of the stove and leave it there all day.

—◊◊—

A full catalog of Italian cooking techniques could fill its own large volume, but this handful is all you will need to prepare any kind of food appropriately and well—and do so efficiently, with an eye toward maximizing nutrition. As you can see, Italians devote the same care and appreciation to the preparation of their food as they do to the eating of it. To my mind, that's all a part of the healthier relationship with food we Americans should learn from them—and key to reaching and maintaining your ideal weight as well as overall good health. It goes hand in hand with tuning back into food, real food, in a way we seem to have forgotten somewhere between Renaissance Tuscany and twenty-first-century America. You're now officially ready to begin your journey. With your cooking techniques refreshed and your pantry and your kitchen stocked, you're all set to put The Diet Code into practice. The final two chapters, with Diet Code menu plans and recipes, will guide you in doing just that.

CHAPTER NINE

The Diet Code Menu Plans

That which chiefly causes the failure of a dinner party is the running short—not of meat, nor yet of drink—but of conversation.

—LEWIS CARROLL

I'll tell you who will end in Hell: . . . teachers of mathematics . . . cats and financiers . . . those who get up early in the morning when they don't have to. Instead, those who will go to Paradise are: . . . Cooks and railroad men, Russians and inventors, wine-tasters . . .

—PRIMO LEVI, FROM *ANOTHER MONDAY*

Now your kitchen is stocked and your stove all but fired up. So what's for dinner? In this chapter, you'll find a variety of menu plans to answer that question for you. Menus for Apprentices, Journeymen or Masters—or vegans, or those feeding a six-year-old, too, or those in serious athletic training or those bent on carving off weight as fast as possible (but still safely). The Diet Code flexes to the requirements of whoever uses it, and though I can't give every permutation here, these basic menu plans will get you started. You can follow these menu plans to the letter, but you'll more likely use them as a springboard to create your own. Mix and match to suit your tastes, your family's preferences, what's in season, the time available to you and what you have on hand. Feel free to draw on menu plans designed for a different phase than your own. There's nothing wrong with eating a vegan meal even if you are a confirmed carnivore, or choosing foods that are surefire hits with kids even if yours are grown and gone, or eating as a Master does when you are just starting out. You may have to adjust some serving sizes, but with all you've learned so far, you should be well prepared to do so. I hope you'll look through all the sections before focusing on the one most immediately suited to you.

Many of these menu plans incorporate dishes you'll find recipes for in chapter 10; those are marked with an asterisk (*). You will find more ideas for complete Diet Code meals in that chapter as well, since many of the recipes are prefaced with serving suggestions for creating well-balanced Diet Code meals.

I've broken down the calorie, carbohydrate, protein and fat content of some of these menu plans for you so you can see exactly how they conform to the Golden Ratio. You will notice that, just the way phi approaches (but will never hit exactly) a 1.1618 value, these meals come close to creating phi without hitting a bull's-eye. Giving yourself about 10% wiggle room on any of the values won't interfere with the effectiveness of the program. Besides, as I demonstrate specifically with the Journeyman menus, as long as you are using a variety of whole foods, the numbers tend to average out over the course of several days anyway.

APPRENTICE MENU PLANS

You don't need to count calories as an Apprentice, but you should be developing an awareness of calorie content, so I've provided them for six menu plans here—three for a target weight of 130 pounds and three for a target weight of 160 pounds—along with the amounts of macronutrients so you can see how they go together to form Golden Ratios.

These menus are designed for the "average woman" and the "average man" (as if there were such people in real life)—someone at, or striving to be at, about 130 pounds who needs 1,950 calories a day, and someone at, or striving to be at, about 160 pounds who needs 2,400 calories a day. Men and women can follow either one—everyone should determine how many calories to include in their diet based on the weight they want to reach (as described in chapter 7). Of course, this isn't one (or even two)-size-fits-all. Naturally, not everyone will be aiming for exactly 1,950 or 2,400 calories a day, but these menu plans will provide a starting point. Consult the Quick Fixes section for adding 100, 150 or 200 calories to a day's menus. Use them as building blocks to shape the calorie counts you want while maintaining a Golden Ratio of macronutrients.

Following the menu plans with complete nutritional breakdowns, you'll find a week's worth of simple suggested menus in a much less precise format suited to the Apprentice. Consult The Diet Code Serving Sizes chart (repeated from chapter 7) to size your portions. Or, use the one-two-three strategy, twice as much protein as grain, three times as much vegetable as grain.

Target: 130 Pounds

For those of you keeping score, the average value for the three days below—1,931 calories, 242 grams of carbs, 98 grams of protein and 61 grams of fat—is very close to The Diet Code Golden Profile Target for 130 pounds: 1,950 calories, 254 grams of carbs, 97 grams of protein and 60 grams of fat. One thing I want you to learn from these menu plans is that even when individual days depart somewhat from the ideal Golden Ratio, over time, the macronutrients tend to balance out as long as you are choosing mainly Fundamental Foods. These menu plans also demonstrate how your two minimeals can be used in different ways, sometimes as snacks and sometimes as dessert after supper.

DAY 1 (TARGET: 130 POUNDS)

	Cal	C	P	F
			grams	
BREAKFAST				
2 oz soft Polenta*	200	38	7	3
4 oz cottage cheese	120	2	21	3
6 oz blueberries	100	22	1	–
1 tbsp honey	68	17	–	–
SNACK				
1 oz Fontina	110	1	7	9
1½ oz dried apricots	116	28	–	–
LUNCH				
4 oz grilled chicken sausage	110	3	12	5
6 oz Braised Broccolini*	150	13	–	9
8 oz Borlotti alla Boscaiolo (Rustic Chili)*	225	40	14	1
SUPPER				
4 oz BBQ turkey kabob	186	–	25	9
6 oz Zucchini al Forno (Oven-Roasted Zucchini)*	150	13	–	9
8 oz corn on the cob	225	40	7	–
DESSERT				
1 oz dark chocolate	100	–	–	11
1¼ oz dried cherries	116	28	1	–
Actual Totals	1,891	245	95	59
Perfect Golden Ratio	1,950	254	97	60

DAY 2 (TARGET: 130 POUNDS)

	Cal	C	P	F
		——grams——		
BREAKFAST				
2 oz tropical granola	200	38	7	3
6 oz banana slices	100	22	1	–
8 oz yogurt	132	13	8	5
SNACK				
1 oz peanut butter	190	7	8	16
6 oz apple slices	100	22	1	–
1 tbsp honey	68	17	–	–
LUNCH				
2 oz multigrain bread	200	38	7	3
4 oz deli-sliced turkey (with roast peppers and fresh basil leaf)	186	–	25	9
6 oz Insalata di Cavolo (Cabbage Salad)*	150	13	–	9
SNACK				
1 oz mixed olives	45	–	–	5
2 oz sesame crackers	200	38	7	3
SUPPER				
4 oz haddock, broiled (with 2 tbsp sweet Thai chili sauce)	120	–	21	2
6 oz Grilled Zucchini*	150	13	–	9
8 oz baked potato	225	40	14	–
Actual Totals	2,066	261	99	64
Perfect Golden Ratio	1,950	254	97	60

DAY 3 (TARGET: 130 POUNDS)

	Cal	C	P	F
		grams		
BREAKFAST				
2 poached eggs	186	–	16	9
6 oz Braised Spinach*	150	13	–	9
8 oz (1 c) black beans	225	40	14	1
SNACK				
1 oz hard Italian cheese	100	1	7	9
6 oz pear slices	100	22	1	–
LUNCH				
2 oz bulgur wheat	200	38	7	3
(with lemon and parsley)				
4 oz white tuna	160	–	26	3
6 oz tomato and avocado salad	150	13	–	9
SUPPER				
5 oz wine	106	2	–	–
4 oz Grilled Devil's Shrimp*	133	–	22	6
6 oz snow peas/leeks	150	13	–	9
DESSERT				
Baked apple:				
6 oz apple	100	22	1	–
2 oz granola	200	38	7	3
1 tbsp honey	68	17	–	–
Actual Totals	1,837	221	101	61
Perfect Golden Ratio	1,950	254	97	60

Target: 160 Pounds

These three days' worth of menus average out to 2,400 calories, 303 grams of carbs, 119 grams of protein and 73 grams of fat—right on point for the perfect Golden Ratio of 2,400 calories, 313 grams of carbs, 120 grams of protein and 74 grams of fat.

DAY 1 (Target: 160 pounds)

	Cal	C	P	F
			grams	
BREAKFAST				
2 oz (avg.) whole wheat English muffin	141	27	6	1
4 oz (3 medium) eggs scrambled with	167	2	15	11
6 oz (1 c) bell peppers	125	10	1	9
6 oz (large) orange	76	18	1	—
SNACK				
4 oz (½ c) cottage cheese	120	2	21	3
6 oz (1¼ c) pineapple	80	19	1	—
LUNCH				
4 oz baked ham slices	200	3	20	12
6 oz (1 c) braised carrots	104	13	4	4
8 oz (1 c) kidney beans	225	40	14	1
6 oz (large) apple	100	25	—	—
SNACK				
2 oz (2 ⅜-inch slices) multigrain bread	190	38	5	2
2 tbsp peanut butter	192	5	8	16
1 tbsp honey	68	17	—	—
SUPPER				
4 oz Tacchino Arrosto (Roast Turkey Thighs)*	172	—	25	8
6 oz (1½ c) Braised Broccoli*	76	7	3	4
8 oz (1 c) corn	212	46	7	—
12 oz beer	146	13	—	—
Actual Totals	2,394	285	131	71
Perfect Golden Ratio	2,400	313	120	74

DAY 2 (TARGET: 160 POUNDS)

	Cal	C	P	F
			grams	
BREAKFAST				
2 oz (1 c cooked) oatmeal	190	35	5	3
6 oz (large) banana	108	26	1	–
8 oz (1 c) yogurt	133	13	9	5
1 tbsp honey	68	17	–	–
SNACK				
¼ c hazelnuts	170	4	7	14
¼ c dried currants	116	28	1	–
LUNCH				
2 oz (3½-inch piece) baguette	190	38	5	2
4 oz sausage	131	3	15	7
6 oz (1 c) Braised Chard*	117	16	4	4
8 oz (1 c) white or cannellini beans	225	40	14	1
SNACK				
2 oz whole rye crackers	190	38	5	2
1 oz (8–10) olives	45	–	–	5
1 oz cheese	109	–	7	9
SUPPER				
4 oz pepper-crusted seared tuna	136	–	25	4
6 oz Grilled Zucchini and Leeks*	81	16	4	–
8 oz (1 c) whipped sweet potatoes with ½ tbsp butter	315	51	3	11
DESSERT				
2 oz (½ c) gelato	133	15	2	7
Actual Totals	2,457	340	107	74
Perfect Golden Ratio	2,400	313	120	74

DAY 3 (TARGET: 160 POUNDS)

	Cal	C	P	F
			grams	
BREAKFAST				
2 oz Bisteca di Pane (Bread Steak)*	208	38	5	4
1 hard-boiled egg	64	1	6	4
2 oz smoked salmon	129	–	12	9
6 oz Grilled Tomatoes*	80	10	1	4
SNACK				
6 oz (1 c) blueberries	104	25	1	–
8 oz (1 c) yogurt	133	13	9	5
LUNCH				
2 oz (¾–1 c cooked) penne pasta	211	40	6	3
4 oz (2 medium) meatballs	278	4	25	18
6 oz (1 c) Sugo al Pomodoro (Simplest Tomato Sauce)*	88	11	2	4
1 tbsp Parmesan	23	–	2	2
SNACK				
2 oz (⅓ c) date-nut granola	200	38	7	3
SUPPER				
2 oz (1 c cooked) rice	203	38	6	3
4 oz red snapper	120	–	21	4
8 oz black beans	225	40	14	1
8 oz Grilled Eggplant* with parsley	137	12	2	9
12 oz beer	146	13	–	–
Actual Totals	2,349	283	120	73
Perfect Golden Ratio	2,400	313	120	74

DRINK

No matter which menu plan you are following, choose your drinks wisely. Have 8 to 13 ounces of liquid at or before each meal—a total of between 1 and 1.5 quarts each day. Your best bets are calorie-free (or all but): water; green, red, white, black or herbal tea; broth or miso—all of which bring nutritional benefits of their own without contributing anything you really don't want in your body (like the high-fructose corn syrup or artificial sweeteners common in so many popular beverages). Espresso and coffee with just a splash of cream fit The Diet Code, too, without really changing the balance of macronutrients. Roasted-grain coffee substitutes alkalize the body and can work as well.

You'll see in some of the menu plans in this chapter that caloric drinks can be worked into the program as well. But avoid sodas, sports drinks and "juices" not made entirely from real fruit—they've got more sugar than vitamins. Red wine and beer are included, of course, and bring health benefits of their own (in—do I even have to say it?—moderation). They are dehydrating, though, so they don't really count in terms of getting your body the fluid it needs. But you can fit in the occasional natural soda or fresh-squeezed orange juice the same way. The important thing is to accommodate them. Just as with dessert, you need to take out calories elsewhere to make room for the calories you drink.

More Apprentice Menu Plans

Use the guidelines here, repeated from The Diet Code Serving Sizes chart and Hand-y Measurements table in chapter 7, to guide your estimates of how much of each food group should be on your plate at each of the meals described below.

APPRENTICE
FIVE FOOD GROUPS SERVING SIZES

FP/fatty protein (cheese, nuts, seeds, nut butter, olives, avocado): 1–2 ounces

G/grains (whole grain bread, pasta, cereal, whole grains): 2 ounces

LP/lean protein (fish, poultry, meat, tempeh, eggs, cottage cheese): 4 ounces

VF/vegetables and fruits (greens, tomatoes, peppers): 6 ounces

SP/starchy proteins (potatoes, beans, peas, corn, yogurt): 8 ounces

HAND-Y MEASUREMENTS

Use your *thumb* to size up rich foods, like cheese and nut butters.

Use *four fingers* to measure a slice of bread.

Use your *cupped hand* to measure dry whole grains, like rice, oatmeal or bulgur, or snack foods like nuts, chips and dried fruit.

Use your *palm* to gauge proteins, like meat, fish, tempeh and (whole) eggs.

Use your *fist* to measure fruits and vegetables; potatoes, beans or yogurt, or cooked pasta or rice.

Monday

BREAKFAST
1 Meini* or other cornbread spread with mascarpone cheese and
   comb honey
Orange sections

SNACK
Pumpkin seeds and golden raisins

LUNCH
Cavolata (Cabbage and Pasta Soup)*

SNACK
Green olives with sesame-wheat breadsticks

SUPPER
Duck breast with marsala glaze
Orzo pasta
Grilled Baby Bok Choi*
Anise gelato

Tuesday

BREAKFAST
Whole grain teff porridge with kefir or soy milk, sliced banana,
   raw sugar and crushed Brazil nuts

LUNCH
Deli-sliced imported sopressata salami in a whole wheat pita with
   tomato and onion slices and romaine
Champagne grapes

SNACK
Pear with pistachios

SUPPER
Roman Fish Soup*
Glass of white wine or beer

DESSERT
Budino (Chocolate Pudding)⋆

Wednesday

BREAKFAST
Yogurt and sliced nectarines with honey, hazelnuts and cardamom

SNACK
Natural sports or nutrition bar

LUNCH
Panzanella (Bread Salad)⋆
Smoked mackerel with lemon wedges

SNACK
Pecans and dried apples

SUPPER
Brodo Miso (Miso Broth)⋆ with dark miso and mushrooms
Spade di Manzo (Skewered Short Ribs)⋆
Mashed potatoes with celeriac
Salad of dandelion greens, white onions, dried cranberries and
    fresh oregano
Glass of red wine or beer

Thursday

BREAKFAST
Micro Meal⋆ (polenta, eggs and greens)

LUNCH
Insalata alla Napoletana (Neapolitan Cauliflower Salad)⋆
Cold sliced roast lamb
Tangerine and Fontina cheese

SNACK
Nicolletta (Hasty Bread Pudding)*

SUPPER
Pesce al Cartoccio (Fish Baked in Parchment)* made with
haddock

DESSERT
Torta Contadina (Rum Raisin Country Cake)*

Friday

BREAKFAST
Whole meal bread with sunflower butter and banana

LUNCH
Cassoeula (Pork Sausage Casserole)*
Sparkling orange beverage

SNACK
Calmyrna figs and Bel Paese soft cheese

SUPPER
Brodo Miso (Miso Broth)* with light miso and slivered red chili
Gamberi Brace alla Diavolo (Grilled Devil's Shrimp)*
Pantacce pasta
Warm green bean salad with artichoke hearts and Walnut White
Wine Dressing*
Glass of white wine or beer

DESSERT
Torrone di Sardegna (Almond Nougat)*

Saturday

BREAKFAST
Frittata* with two eggs and asparagus
Mimosa (Italian-style, with Prosecco)

LUNCH

Pizza margherita with crushed tomato, fresh mozzarella and basil leaf

Chinotto bitter orange beverage

SNACK

Grapefruit sections drizzled with lime blossom honey

SUPPER

Agnello All 'Aceto (Lamb Stew)*

Mixed root vegetables

DESSERT

Brutti ("Ugly" Meringues)*

Espresso

SUNDAY BRUNCH

I love to indulge in a big brunch on Sunday, basically combining a breakfast and a midmorning snack (or a snack and a lunch) into one larger meal. My favorite is an antipasti spread of by now familiar Golden Ratio foods:

 1 oz (8–10) brine-cured olives
 1 oz ricotta salata cheese
 2 oz (2 ⅜-inch slices of a 4-inch-square loaf) whole meal bread
 2 oz smoked salmon
 1 hard-boiled egg
 3 oz (⅓ c) Caponata (Sweet and Sour Eggplant)*
 3 oz (⅔ c) tomato and green onion salad
 Lemon wedges
 Coffee

JOURNEYMAN MENU PLANS

These six days' worth of menu plans are also designed for people targeting 130 and 160 pounds. This time, the basic meals and snacks are mostly the same between the two plans, but with additional snacks or servings figured into the higher calorie count (listed in boldface type). Whichever plan you are closer to yourself, it will be instructive to take note of some of the ways an additional 450 calories fits into a diet. In one case, it's not much more than adding dessert. Think about what that means for someone who hasn't accommodated that sort of thing into their program and is eating dessert every day anyway. It wouldn't take long for those additions to add up to some significant excess poundage. Just one soda a day—150 calories—could create about 15 extra pounds a year.

Here again I've intentionally varied the nutritional breakdowns somewhat over the week—higher in protein on some days, higher in fat or carbs on others. I want you to see that over the full cycle of menus (taking the 130-pound plan as an example) you get pretty close to that Golden Ratio target of 1,950 calories (130 × 15), 254 grams of carb, 97 grams of protein, 60 grams of fat. These plans assume you are using foods with their natural fat contents (full-fat dairy, poultry with skin, meats trimmed but with about ⅛ inch of visible fat intact) and dressing vegetables with 1 teaspoon of olive oil.

Target: 130 Pounds

MONDAY (TARGET: 130 POUNDS)

	Cal	C	P	F
		grams		
BREAKFAST	450	50	22	18
1 Alpine Baked Porridge Muffin*				
8 oz (1 c) buttermilk or kvass				
SNACK	282	32	7	14
¼ c almonds				
¼ c dried papaya				
LUNCH	453	44	31	17
1 c chickpea Miso Broth*				
2 sprouted-grain tortillas				
Chunky salad:				
¼ avocado, ½ 6-oz can tuna,				
¾ c tomato wedges, scallions and parsley				
2 tsp Lemon Caper Dressing*				
SNACK	152	17	12	4
3 oz (⅓ c) cottage cheese				
5 oz (¾) sliced peaches				
SUPPER	464	51	25	6
2 oz (3-inch) rustic baguette				
1½–2 c Minestra di Pesce				
(Seafood Soup)*				
5 oz wine				
DESSERT	152	38	–	–
5 oz (1 c) blackberries				
1 tbsp lime blossom honey				
Actual Totals	1,953	232	97	59
Perfect Golden Ratio	1,950	254	97	60

Target: 160 Pounds

MONDAY (Target: 160 Pounds)

	Cal	C	P	F
		grams		
BREAKFAST 1 Alpine Baked Porridge Muffin★ 8 oz (1 c) buttermilk or kvass	450	50	22	18
SNACK ¼ c almonds ¼ c dried papaya	282	32	7	14
LUNCH 1 c chickpea Miso Broth★ 2 sprouted-grain tortillas Chunky salad: ¼ avocado, ½ 6-oz can tuna, ¾ c tomato wedges, scallions and parsley 2 tsp Lemon Caper Dressing★	453	44	31	17
SNACK 3 oz (⅓ c) cottage cheese 5 oz (¾ c) sliced peaches	152	17	12	4
SUPPER 2 oz (3-inch) rustic baguette 1½–2 c Minestra di Pesce (Seafood Soup)★ **made with 2 additional ounces of fish** **12 oz beer**	557	62	36	7
DESSERT 5 oz (1 c) blackberries 1 tbsp lime blossom honey **¼ c ricotta cheese** **Sbriciolona (Crumb Cookie)★**	507	86	12	13
Actual Totals	2,401	291	120	73
Perfect Golden Ratio	2,400	313	120	74

TUESDAY (Target: 130 Pounds)

	Cal	C	P	F
		grams		
Breakfast	233	37	10	5
1 c yogurt				
5 oz (¾ c) blueberries, warmed with				
lemon zest, ground nutmeg or mace and:				
1 tsp raw sugar				
Snack	228	40	8	4
2 oz (⅓ c) maple-nut granola				
Lunch	404	41	24	16
1 c barley Miso Broth*				
2 oz Bavarian-style bread				
2 hard-boiled eggs made into				
egg salad dressed with:				
1 tbsp Caesar dressing*				
5 oz Braised Dandelion Greens*				
Snack	197	31	7	5
5 oz (1 medium) banana				
1 c soy milk				
Supper	468	53	28	16
3 oz Pollo ai Limoni (Lemon Chicken)*				
5 oz (1 c) Braised Green Beans*				
garnished with:				
1 tbsp toasted almond flakes				
8 oz (1 medium) baked russet potato served with:				
1 tbsp sour cream				
Dessert	339	57	12	7
Budino (Chocolate Pudding)*				
5 oz (¾ c) strawberries pureed				
with orange zest and:				
1 tsp raw sugar				
Actual Totals	1,869	259	89	53
Perfect Golden Ratio	1,950	254	97	60

TUESDAY (TARGET: 160 POUNDS)

	Cal	C	P	F
		grams		
BREAKFAST	461	77	18	9
1 c yogurt				
5 oz (¾ c) blueberries, warmed with lemon zest, ground nutmeg or mace and:				
1 tsp raw sugar				
2 oz (⅓ c) maple-nut granola				
SNACK	197	31	7	5
5 oz (1 medium) banana				
1 c soy milk				
LUNCH	547	45	31	27
1 c barley Miso Broth*				
2 oz Bavarian-style bread				
3 hard-boiled eggs made into egg salad dressed with:				
1 tbsp Caesar dressing*				
¼ fruit avocado				
5 oz Braised Dandelion Greens*				
SNACK	384	52	21	10
2 oz (2 6-inch) corn tortillas				
3 oz bacon-wrapped scallops (½ oz bacon, 1 strip)				
1 (medium) green apple, sliced				
SUPPER	468	53	28	16
3 oz Pollo ai Limoni (Lemon Chicken)*				
5 oz (1 c) Braised Green Beans* garnished with:				
1 tbsp toasted almond flakes				
8 oz (1 medium) baked russet potato served with:				
1 tbsp sour cream				
DESSERT	339	57	12	7
Budino (Chocolate Pudding)*				
5 oz (¾ c) strawberries pureed with orange zest and:				
1 tsp raw sugar				
Actual Totals	2,396	315	117	74
Perfect Golden Ratio	2,400	313	120	74

WEDNESDAY (TARGET: 130 POUNDS)

	Cal	C	P	F
		grams		
BREAKFAST	341	57	8	9

2 oz dry (1 c cooked) hot brown rice cereal with:
¼ c half and half
1 tbsp maple syrup

SNACK	88	2	11	4

3 oz (⅓ c) cottage cheese

LUNCH	441	57	24	13

2 oz (2 6-inch) corn tortillas for fajitas with:
4 oz Grilled Tempeh*
2 tbsp Crema di Carciofi (Creamy Artichoke Dip)*
5 oz (1 c) diced fresh tomato, red onion and bell peppers

SNACK	241	8	23	13

3 oz lobster cocktail
5 oz (1 c) celery sticks filled with:
1 oz gorgonzola cheese

SUPPER	525	56	37	17

1 c soybean Miso Broth*
3 oz grilled lamb sirloin
5 oz (1 c) braised carrots, parsnips and turnips
  with coriander, turmeric and:
1 tsp olive oil
8 oz (1 c) black beluga lentils with marjoram

DESSERT	320	55	7	8

Fichi Pignati (Poached Figs)* served over:
¼ c ricotta

	Cal	C	P	F
Actual Totals	1,956	235	110	64
Perfect Golden Ratio	1,950	254	97	60

WEDNESDAY (TARGET: 160 POUNDS)

	Cal	C	P	F
			grams	
BREAKFAST	540	87	12	16
2 oz dry (1 c cooked) hot brown rice cereal with:				
¼ c half and half				
1 tbsp maple syrup				
2 tbsp almond flakes				
¼ c chopped prunes				
SNACK	140	14	12	4
3 oz (⅓ c) cottage cheese				
5 oz (1 c) nectarine slices				
LUNCH	441	57	24	13
2 oz (2 6-inch) corn tortillas for fajitas with:				
4 oz Grilled Tempeh*				
2 tbsp Crema di Carciofi (Creamy Artichoke Dip)*				
5 oz (1 c) diced fresh tomato, red onion and bell peppers				
SNACK	241	8	23	13
3 oz lobster cocktail				
5 oz (1 c) celery sticks filled with:				
1 oz gorgonzola cheese				
SUPPER	715	94	42	179
1 c soybean Miso Broth*				
3 oz grilled lamb sirloin				
5 oz (1 c) braised carrots, parsnips and				
turnips with coriander, turmeric and:				
1 tsp olive oil				
8 oz (1 c) black beluga lentils with marjoram				
2 oz dry (1 c cooked) couscous				
DESSERT	320	55	7	8
Fichi Pignati (Poached Figs)* served over:				
¼ c ricotta				
Actual Totals	2,397	315	120	73
Perfect Golden Ratio	2,400	313	120	74

THURSDAY (TARGET: 130 POUNDS)

	Cal	C	P	F
		grams		
BREAKFAST	359	45	20	11
2 oz dry (¾ c cooked) Polenta* topped with:				
2 eggs, poached				
5 oz (¾ c) green salsa				
1 tbsp grated Parmesan				
SNACK	201	30	9	5
1 c yogurt				
1 tbsp amarena (sour cherry) fruit preserves				
LUNCH	528	77	19	16
1 c white rice Miso Broth*				
2 oz (2 6-inch) sprouted-grain tortillas				
4 oz (½ c) black bean spread				
5 oz (¾ c) roasted red pepper and white onion salad				
SNACK	222	16	8	14
2 oz (¼ c) walnuts				
5 oz (¾ c) honeydew melon				
SUPPER	522	60	30	18
Halibut alla Pizzaiola (Halibut Pizza Style)*				
2 oz dry (1 c cooked) couscous				
5 oz (1 c) Braised Broccolini* with:				
Lemon wedges				
DESSERT	193	21	7	81
1 oz cheese				
5 oz (1 medium) pear				
Actual Totals	2,025	249	93	73
Perfect Golden Ratio	1,950	254	97	60

THURSDAY (TARGET: 160 POUNDS)

	Cal	C	P	F
			grams	
BREAKFAST 2 oz dry (¾ c cooked) Polenta* topped with: 2 eggs, poached 5 oz (¾ c) green salsa 1 tbsp grated Parmesan **8 oz (1 c) kvass**	457	57	28	13
SNACK 1 c yogurt 1 tbsp amarena (sour cherry) fruit preserves **5 oz (2 medium) kiwi**	301	54	10	5
LUNCH 1 c white rice Miso Broth* 2 oz (2 6-inch) sprouted-grain tortillas 4 oz (½ c) black bean spread 5 oz (¾ c) roasted red pepper and white onion salad **3 oz crabmeat**	596	77	36	16
SNACK 2 oz (¼ c) walnuts 5 oz (¾ c) honeydew melon	222	16	8	14
SUPPER Halibut alla Pizzaiola (Halibut Pizza Style)* 2 oz dry (1 c cooked) couscous 5 oz (1 c) Braised Broccolini* with: Lemon wedges **5 oz wine**	628	62	30	18
DESSERT 1 oz cheese 5 oz (1 medium) pear	193	21	7	81
Actual Totals	2,397	287	119	75
Perfect Golden Ratio	2,400	313	120	74

FRIDAY (TARGET: 130 POUNDS)

	Cal	C	P	F
			grams	
BREAKFAST	405	64	17	9
2 oz dry (1 c cooked) bulgur wheat				
1 c kefir				
1 tbsp raw sugar				
SNACK	68	17	–	–
5 oz (2 medium) plums				
LUNCH	428	48	23	16
2 oz (1 c cooked) angel hair pasta with				
vodka sauce and scallions, parsley and:				
2 oz scallops				
1 oz black caviar				
5 oz (¾ c) Asparagi Grigliata (Grilled Asparagus)*				
SNACK	140	14	12	4
3 oz (⅓ c) cottage cheese				
5 oz (¾ c) cantaloupe				
SUPPER	612	52	34	18
1 c chickpea Miso Broth*				
2 oz dry (1 c cooked) brown and wild rice				
3 oz grilled center-cut pork chop glazed with:				
1 tsp orange marmalade				
1 tsp rum				
5 oz (¾ c) Braised Snow Peas* and scallions				
5 oz wine				
DESSERT	308	47	12	8
8 oz (1 c) pumpkin custard (crustless				
pie filling baked in a ramekin)				
Actual Totals	1,961	242	98	55
Perfect Golden Ratio	1,950	254	97	60

FRIDAY (TARGET: 160 POUNDS)

	Cal	C	P	F
		grams		
BREAKFAST	521	92	18	9
2 oz dry (1 c cooked) bulgur wheat				
1 c kefir				
1 tbsp raw sugar				
¼ c raisins				
SNACK	68	17	–	–
5 oz (2 medium) plums				
LUNCH	428	48	23	16
2 oz (1 c cooked) angel hair pasta with				
vodka sauce and scallions, parsley and:				
2 oz scallops				
1 oz black caviar				
5 oz (¾ c) Asparagi Grigliata (Grilled Asparagus)*				
SNACK	140	14	12	4
3 oz (⅓ c) cottage cheese				
5 oz (¾ c) cantaloupe				
SUPPER	728	60	46	22
1 c chickpea Miso Broth*				
2 oz dry (1 c cooked) brown and wild rice				
3 oz grilled center-cut pork chop glazed with:				
1 tsp orange marmalade				
1 tsp rum				
5 oz (¾ c) Braised Snow Peas* and scallions				
5 oz wine				
12 medium oysters				
DESSERT	503	52	22	23
8 oz (1 c) pumpkin custard (crustless pie filling baked in a ramekin)				
2 oz (⅓ c) ricotta				
½ oz (2 tbsp) crushed walnuts				
Actual Totals	2,388	280	121	74
Perfect Golden Ratio	2,400	313	120	74

SATURDAY (TARGET: 130 POUNDS)

	Cal	C	P	F
		grams		
BREAKFAST	468	60	21	16
6 Crespelle (Buckwheat Crepes)* layered with:				
2 tbsp sour cream				
1 tbsp raw sugar				
SNACK	92	22	1	—
8 oz (1 c) black grapes				
LUNCH	527	63	35	15
1 c white rice Miso Broth*				
2 oz dry (¾–1 c cooked) orecchiette pasta				
3 oz grilled bluefish				
5 oz (¾ c) fresh peas sautéed with minced onion and mint				
SNACK	64	15	—	—
5 oz (1 large) orange				
SUPPER	560	58	28	24
3 oz Chianti-glazed chicken breast				
5 oz (¾ c) ratatouille (zucchini, tomato and onion ragout)				
8 oz (¾ c) fresh corn				
DESSERT	224	33	10	5
1 c yogurt				
5 oz (1 c) raspberries				
1 tsp raw sugar				
Actual Totals	1,935	251	95	60
Perfect Golden Ratio	1,950	254	97	60

SATURDAY (Target: 160 Pounds)

	Cal	C	P	F
			grams	
Breakfast	651	74	32	25
6 Crespelle (Buckwheat Crepes)* layered with:				
2 tbsp sour cream				
1 tbsp raw sugar				
½ oz (2 tbsp) cracked hazelnuts				
8 oz (1 c) buttermilk				
Snack	92	22	1	–
8 oz (1 c) black grapes				
Lunch	527	63	35	15
1 c white rice Miso Broth*				
2 oz dry (¾–1 c cooked) orecchiette pasta				
3 oz grilled bluefish				
5 oz (¾ c) fresh peas sautéed with minced onion and mint				
Snack	64	15	–	–
5 oz (1 large) orange				
Supper	821	98	42	29
3 oz Chianti-glazed chicken breast				
5 oz (¾ c) ratatouille (zucchini, tomato and onion ragout)				
8 oz (¾ c) fresh corn				
8 oz (1 c) lima beans				
Dessert	224	33	10	5
1 c yogurt				
5 oz (1 c) raspberries				
1 tsp raw sugar				
Actual Totals	2,379	305	120	74
Perfect Golden Ratio	2,400	313	120	74

Quick Fixes

No matter what stage of The Diet Code you are in or which menu plans you are following, there are two fast and easy ways to adjust any one of the menus given in this chapter to the exact calorie count you've chosen for yourself without compromising the Golden Ratio of macronutrients. Your first option is to proportionally change the serving size of any of The Diet Code dishes. You know the meals are balanced, so you know they'll stay in balance as you serve yourself a little more or a little less than is specified in a menu plan. One caution: For the most part, these will be small changes, measured in ounces and tablespoons. Don't take it as license to double your servings! Your macronutrients might still be in Golden Proportion, but your calories will quickly get out of line.

The other strategy is to choose among the following Quick Fixes, adding them to a snack or meal. Select something complementary to the meal or snack you're adding to. If the scheduled snack is just grapes, choose cottage cheese, for example, to add protein and fat to the grapes' carbs. Note that yogurt and kefir are naturally the most balanced foods and come as close as any of food can to hitting the Golden Ratio. On the chart, I've included one type of prepared food—two specific energy bars made from whole, natural foods that give you the macronutrients in nearly the Golden Ratio—the quickest (and simplest) Quick Fix of all.

100 CALORIES

Serving Size	Dominant Macronutrients
¾ oz chocolate	fat
3 oz light/white fish	protein
1 oz cheese	protein and fat
⅓ c cottage cheese	carbs, protein and fat*
1 c vegetables dressed with 1 tsp olive oil	carbs and fat
1 medium–large piece of fruit	carbs
5-oz glass of wine	carbs**

150 CALORIES

Serving Size	Dominant Macronutrients
3 oz poultry	protein and fat
3 oz sardines	protein and fat
8 oz (1 c) yogurt or kefir	carbs, protein and fat*
2 6-inch sprouted-grain tortillas	carbs
12 oz beer	carbs

200 CALORIES

Serving Size	Dominant Macronutrients
Handful of nuts	protein and fat
2 oz (¾–1 c cooked) pasta	carbs and protein
1 large potato	carbs and protein
1 large ear corn	carbs and protein
Greens+ Natural Energy Bar or Zoe's Flax and Soy Bar	carbs, protein and fat***

GOLDEN COMBINATIONS***

Serving Size	Calories
8 oz (1 c) yogurt and ½ c berries	170
4 oz (½ c) beans with 1 oz cheese melted on top	220
2 oz (4–8) whole grain crackers with 2 oz smoked salmon	330
2 oz whole grain toast (2 ⅜-inch slices) and 2 eggs	340
Baker's lunch (3 oz whole grain or artisanal sourdough bread, 1 oz aged Asiago cheese, ½ oz [6 filets] white anchovies)	372

* Contains all three macronutrients, but too evenly distributed to create the Golden Ratio.

** Though it does contain some carbs, most of the calories in wine actually come from the alcohol itself, which is not a macronutrient.

*** Golden!

MASTER MENU PLAN

One of the hallmarks of being a Diet Code Master is that you're not using menu plans someone else put together for you anymore. But I do keep a list posted on my fridge of meals I know I like to make and eat—and that my kids like—to make sure I keep them in regular rotation without falling into any particular ruts. And of course, the way you'll develop your personally tailored menus is by trying out, and then adjusting, various menu plans. So for what it's worth, here's the basic itinerary of my personal Diet Code. I use it to maintain my weight at about 160 pounds in portions that yield 2,400 calories, with 313 grams of carbs, 120 grams of protein and 74 grams of fat.

Upon waking
Miso Broth*

Breakfast
Whole grain porridge with apple and kefir
or
Eggs with Polenta* or bread and Braised Greens* or salsa

Snack
Bread, with nut butter or cheese or anchovies

Lunch
Beans (any style) or Caponata* or potato salad
Sausage or hard-boiled egg or tempeh or smoked fish
Sauerkraut or Insalata di Cavolo* or tomato salad or roast peppers
  or kimchi

Snack
Fruit
Nuts

Supper
Pasta or rice or sweet potato
Fresh fish or meat

Asparagus *or* greens *or* squash
    or peas *or* Misticanza*

NIGHT
Yogurt with honey and crushed nuts or seeds

One of the important ways I make The Diet Code my own, so it serves the particular needs of my body, is to cluster more food around my martial arts workouts, about 1,000 extra calories for one *very* intense hour, three times a week. Exercise and diet interlock to optimize metabolism. To get the most out of both, I make sure to get extra fat about an hour before a workout and extra carbs immediately after, along with the protein I always include. With a peanut butter (3 tbsp) and honey (1 tbsp) sandwich on Bavarian-type bread (two ¼-inch slices) before, and a microwaved porridge of barley, spelt and rye flakes (⅔ c dry all together) with flax (1 tbsp), dried fruit (¼ c) and honey or molasses (1 tbsp) served with yogurt (1 c) afterward, I get about 20 grams of protein (body weight × 0.125) before and after. That's 26 grams of fat preworkout and almost 100 grams of carbs postworkout. That's twice the usual proportion of both fat and carbs.

1,500-CALORIE CRUNCH DIET

This 1,500-calorie diet is the bare minimum of calories any adult should ever subsist on (remember that it's only enough to sustain a 100-pound adult over the long term), but it is a fast way to peel off weight. What I'm presenting here is meant to be used for one month only, as a sort of detox program to kick your weight loss into high gear. But even choosing the very best foods at every turn here, it wouldn't be smart to limit your body to this number of calories over any longer a time period than that. Cutting back your calories this far should increase your weight loss rate to about 10 pounds a month. It would be wise to consult with your health care professional before embarking on any drastic regimen, especially if you have existing health issues.

To do this crash program right, you must not cheat yourself nutri-tionally. Eat the best quality, most densely nutritious natural, whole foods—Fundamental Foods—to keep the nutrient level at a premium and to ensure your well-being. You must not cheat yourself of treats, either, so even on this pared-down plan, you'll still make room for the occasional glass of wine or hunk of chocolate. (My nona would come back from the other side if she learned my diet would deny anyone a little vino!) You'll be eating bread and full-fat everything. There are limits to indulgence, though, and you should be aware that a single fast-food stop for just a burger, fries and a drink can easily meet or exceed the entire day's calorie quota.

At the 1,500-calories-per-day level, there is no "day off" after six days on the program. It would be too easy to undo all your hard work on this plan, which doesn't grant as much room to flex as do the others. Other than that, this is essentially a version of the Journey-man plan. You'll eat the Journeyman's six small meals a day, but here you'll get three main meals of about 350 calories each and three small meals of just 150 calories each. This means portions are scaled back to about two-thirds (or 67%) of normal Diet Code portions of 1, 2, 3, 5 and 8 ounces, producing the following serving-size guidelines:

⅔ oz (2 tbsp) cheese or nuts
1⅓ oz dry (⅔ c cooked) pasta or grain
2 oz meat
3⅓ oz (⅓–⅔ c) vegetable or fruit
5⅓ oz (⅔ c) yogurt, beans or potato

For the main and minimeals on the 1,500-calorie program, the macronutrient profile according to the Golden Ratio looks like this:

Cal.	Carbs (g)	Protein (g)	Fat (g)
150	20	7	4.5
350	46	18	11

When your calorie intake is this low, it's more important to keep those figures constant in order to keep your metabolism steady, so

---

MEASURING UP

You can keep your calorie counts more accurate and make life a little easier on yourself by designating a set of measuring spoons and cups specifically for Diet Code foods. For the 1,500-calorie diet, your special set should include a teaspoon, a tablespoon and a ⅓-cup dry measuring cup.

Use the teaspoon for honey and olive oil. Two tablespoons gives you the right amount (65–100 calories worth) of nuts, dried fruit, cheese and sour cream. The ⅓-cup measure portions out dry oatmeal and flaked grains for breakfast cereal (to ⅔ c water). Use it twice to measure cooked pasta, rice and whole grains, beans, mashed potatoes, yogurt, fruit and vegetables.

Oh, and set aside a special small wineglass as well, 4 to 5 ounces in capacity, and fill it using the ⅓-cup measure.

---

these menus are designed to meet the Golden Ratio closely at all times, not relying on averaging out over a few days or a week.

Monday

BREAKFAST
1 Alpine Baked Porridge Muffin*

SNACK
3⅓ oz (⅓ c) mango slices

LUNCH
2 oz (⅓ c) white tuna over:
3⅓ oz (⅔ c) Braised Asparagus* (1 tsp olive oil) served with:
Lemon wedge
5⅓ oz (⅔ c) Ceci alla Sardegna (Sardinian Chickpea Salad)*

SNACK
¾ oz dark chocolate

SUPPER

2 braised stuffed cabbage leaves (filled with:

1 oz ground beef browned with minced onion

⅔ c cooked brown rice

1 tbsp Parmesan)

⅔ c carrots braised (1 tsp olive oil) with:

Parsley

DESSERT

3⅓ oz (⅔ c) cherries

⅓ c wine

Tuesday

BREAKFAST

⅔ c warm Polenta* with honey

3 oz (⅓ c) cottage cheese

3⅓ oz (⅔ c) cantaloupe slices

SNACK

½ oz (2 tbsp) pecans

LUNCH

2 tbsp olives

1½ oz (¼-inch slice) Bavarian-type bread

2 oz smoked salmon

⅔ c Insalata di Cavolo (Cabbage Salad)*

SNACK

1 oz Fontina cheese

3⅓ oz (⅔ c) grapes

SUPPER

Halibut alla Pizzaiola (Halibut Pizza Style)*

⅓ c Polenta*

DESSERT

3⅓ oz (⅔ c) peach slices

2 tbsp cream

Wednesday

BREAKFAST
1 Meini*
1 tbsp 100% fruit preserves
⅔ c buttermilk or soy milk

SNACK
½ oz (2 tbsp) macadamia nuts

LUNCH
2 oz smoked turkey breast (deli sliced) piled on:
1½ oz (¼-inch slice) Bavarian-style bread spread with:
2 tbsp Crema di Carciofi (Creamy Artichoke Dip)* and:
⅓ c roast peppers
⅔ c Acqua Fredda (Italian Gazpacho)*

SNACK
¾ oz dark chocolate

SUPPER
Uova al Piatto (Baked Eggs with Beans and Salsa)*

DESSERT
3⅓ oz (⅔ c) honeydew melon
⅓ c white wine

Thursday

BREAKFAST
2 eggs scrambled with:
½ oz (2 tbsp) shredded cheese and:
Slivered basil over:
3 oz (⅔ c) fresh baby spinach
1 orange

SNACK
½ oz (2 tbsp) pistachios
2 tbsp dried cranberries

LUNCH

Frutti di Mare (seafood salad):

2 oz poached shrimp, 2 oz poached scallops, ⅔ c quinoa rotelle
    pasta, 2⅓ c filet beans, 2 tsp olive oil, lemon juice and parsley

SNACK

5 dates

SUPPER

⅔ c Passata di Zucca (Creamy Squash Soup)⋆

3 oz grilled chicken sausage link

⅔ c Braised Kale⋆ (1 tsp olive oil)

DESSERT

⅔ c blueberries

⅔ c yogurt with:

1 tsp honey

Friday

BREAKFAST

⅔ c cooked oatmeal

⅔ c yogurt with:

1 tsp honey

3⅓ oz (⅓ c) (1 small) banana, sliced

SNACK

½ oz (2 tbsp) cashews

LUNCH

Caprese Sandwich:

1½ oz (¼-inch slice) Bavarian-style bread; arrange alternate
    pieces of:

2 oz fresh mozzarella, sliced

1 large sliced tomato

6 fresh basil leaves

1 tsp olive oil drizzled over layers

SNACK
¾ oz dark chocolate

SUPPER
1⅔ c Minestra di Pesce (Seafood Soup)*
1 (small–medium) ear corn on the cob (*or* ⅔ c corn off the cob)

DESSERT
3⅓ oz (⅔ c) raspberries
1 oz (2 tbsp) ricotta with:
1 tsp honey

Saturday

BREAKFAST
1⅓ oz (⅓ c) granola
3⅓ oz (⅔ c) blackberries
5⅓ oz (⅔ c) yogurt

SNACK
5 dried apricots
½ oz (2 tbsp) almonds

LUNCH
3 oz chicken breast braised in white wine
⅔ c Zucchini al Forno (Oven-Roasted Zucchini)*

SNACK
3⅓ oz (⅔ c) pineapple chunks
½ oz (⅓ c) shredded coconut

SUPPER
2 oz oregano-grilled lamb sirloin
3⅓ (⅔ c) Grilled Brussels Sprouts* with:
1 tsp olive oil
5⅓ oz (⅔ c) potato with:
1 tbsp sour cream and chives

Dessert
2 dried figs
⅓ c red wine

Sunday

Breakfast
Melt the following under broiler:
1 poached egg on:
1 oz sliced capocollo ham and:
1 slab beefsteak tomato on:
1 small whole grain pita, all topped with:
1 oz deli-slice provolone

Snack
3⅓ oz (½ large) pear
⅔ oz (2 tbsp) sweet gorgonzola cheese

Lunch
1⅓ c Zuppa di Lenticce all 'Abruzzese (Lentil Soup)* with:
1 tbsp Parmesan

Snack
¾ oz dark chocolate

Supper
Cozze e Risotto (Mussels and Risotto)*:
    8 oz (1⅓ c) mussels
    3⅓ oz (⅔ c cooked) risotto, with:
    1 tbsp shaved Parmesan
3⅓ oz (1 c) Misticanza (Wild Greens Salad)* with:
1 tbsp dressing

Dessert
3⅓ oz (⅔ c) strawberries
2 tbsp cream

MENU FOR THE MAN OF MUSCLE

Rick comes into Sophia's just about every week. Standing 6 feet, 9 inches tall, he can hardly be expected to live on 2 ounces of grain, 3 ounces of protein and 5 ounces of vegetables. But he can, should and does still eat Golden. He doesn't choose a Da Vinci Plate and then some side dishes. He says the proportions taste so good the way they are that he doesn't want to spoil anything. He just orders double! He inspired me to plan this menu for all the really big boys, scaled up from a 2–3–5–8 Fibonacci progression to a 3–5–8–13 series. The resulting sample menu is for a 220-pound person (or someone aiming to be): 3,300 calories (220 × 15).

BREAKFAST
5 oz (3 large) eggs, fried
8 oz (1½ c) sautéed zucchini and peppers
12 oz (1½ c) white beans with bacon and sage

SNACK
5 oz (⅔ c) cottage cheese
8 oz (2 c) grapes

LUNCH
5 oz grilled trout
8 oz (2 c) Braised Red and Green Cabbage with Fennel*
13 oz (2 c) tortelli pasta stuffed with pumpkin

SNACK
5 oz shrimp cocktail
12 oz beer (There are no 13-oz beers available, but if you want to pop open another bottle for that righteous swig, you'll get no argument from me.)

Supper

5 oz grilled sirloin

8 oz (1½ c) broccoli with seared portobello mushrooms

13 oz (1½ c) lemon thyme roast potatoes

Dessert

1 oz (2 tbsp) sour cream

8 oz (1 c) plums sautéed with cardamom

1 tbsp honey *or* demerara sugar

	Calories	Carbs	Protein	Fat
Actual Totals:	3,283	425 g	166 g	102 g
Golden Profile Target:	3,300	432 g	165 g	101 g

VEGAN MEAL PLANS

Even without meat, fish, shellfish, eggs, milk, cheese or even honey, there's still a lot of possibilities left for your plate. Nevertheless, most vegans I've met (in the decades since I was one myself) don't know how to cook, and instead eat plenty of refined and otherwise processed foods. And they are addicted to sugar. White sugar. Vegans benefit as much as anyone from refocusing on whole, natural foods, albeit solely of the plant variety. Enough with the isolates of this and the hydrolyzed that! Instead, think Fundamental Foods: quinoa, spelt, rice, rye. Black beans, red beans, lentils, chickpeas. Avocado, sunflower butter, walnuts, hemp. Asparagus, kale, broccolini, parsley. Beets, winter squash, sweet potato, tomato sauce. Prunes, figs, melon, berries. Miso, kimchi, nori flakes, tempeh.

The menu plan here delivers 16% of its calories as protein, which is below The Diet Code profile but well within a healthy range. To avoid soy isolate powders and soy-based meat substitutes—fractured foods—I recommend the most potent vegetable protein source on the planet: hemp. Food-grade hemp seed meal has 14 grams of protein per ounce, *three times* that of beef or tuna, the densest animal sources. It's also a great source of omega-3 essential fatty acids. Sprinkle naturally soft shelled hemp seeds on soy "yogurt" or porridges; roll bananas drizzled with fruit syrup in them; add them into whole grain baked goods like Meini or Alpine Baked Porridge Muffins (see recipes on pp. 268 and 269). The green "butter" (like pumpkin-seed butter, another vegan superfood) and fluffy green meal are equally good sources of this premier protein.

The menu plan below is designed for a person aiming at 130 pounds (1,950 calories). For 160 pounds, you need to add another 450 calories. You can increase, in proportion, some serving sizes, or add in a substantial snack. Handily, the fruit and hemp balls described below provide nearly ideal Golden Ratio macronutrient proportions. Grab two to make up the difference easily.

UPON WAKING
1c barley Miso Broth*

BREAKFAST
2 oz (⅓ c) Quinoa Porridge*
1 tbsp almond butter
1½ oz (¼ c) chopped mission figs and prunes

SNACK
8 oz (1 c) soy yogurt
½ oz (2 tbsp) hemp seed

LUNCH
2 oz (2) sprouted-grain pitas
4 oz Grilled Tempeh*
2 tbsp Crema di Carciofi (Creamy Artichoke Dip)*
¼ c roast peppers
5 oz (1 c) Cavolo Nero Brasato (Braised Black Kale)*

SNACK
5 oz (1 c) mixed berries and cantaloupe

SUPPER

5 oz (1 c) Asparagi Grigliata (Grilled Asparagus)* and grilled
    scallions with a seaweed sprinkle
8 oz (1 c) black beans stewed with mushroom
    concentrate
8 oz (1 c) sweet potato
1 tbsp walnut butter

HEMP AND FRUIT BALLS

Cultivated thousands of years ago in Russia and China and once
prized by the founding fathers of this country, hemp is so high in
protein that constructing a perfect Golden Ratio meal around it
requires adding 28 grams of carbohydrates and 4.5 grams of fat
to every ounce of the seed meal. That's ¼ cup of dried fruit and
1 teaspoon of vegetable oil, exactly. So that's precisely what this
recipe does.

- Mash, pound or pulse in a food processor into a shape-
  able paste:
  5 oz hemp seed meal
  5 tsp flax or nut oil
  7½ oz (5 quarter cups or 1¼ c) mixed dried fruit
- Chill, divide evenly into eight pieces, and roll into balls.

Each will have 225 calories, a perfect Diet Code profile (29 grams
of carbs, 11 grams of protein, 7 grams of fat)—and a weight of
about 1.618 ounces!

FAMILY FRIENDLY

The Diet Code is good for the whole family. Since it's an eating plan for life rather than a time-limited crash diet, The Diet Code works as well for children and teenagers as it does for anyone else. Everyone eating at your table can enjoy the same whole, natural foods in simple preparations—no making separate meals for you (or them).

It's always most important to consider what fuels and supports kids' healthy growth. This isn't meant to be a weight loss plan for kids. Like anyone else, however, children on The Diet Code will experience optimal health, and that includes the weight that's right for their rapidly growing bodies. This is to say, make sure you feed your kids *enough*—they need as much or more than adults do. Making sure the food they get is maximally nutrient-rich is even more important in developing bodies. This is no time to be subsisting on chicken nuggets and fruit punch (advertising "10% real juice!").

The National Academy of Sciences, which determines the RDA (Recommended Daily Allowances), suggests that children ages 1 to 3 need 1,300 calories per day; 4- to 6-year-olds need 1,800 calories; kids from 7 to 10 need 2,000 calories; girls between 11 and 14 need 2,200 calories, while boys of the same ages need 2,500 calories. So the preceeding 1,500-calorie menus starting on p. 231 have serving sizes fit for the needs of a 3- to 4-year-old (though a young palate may need some different food choices). The Apprentice or Journeyman plans for a target weight of 130 pounds would approximate what a 7- to 10-year-old needs. A 16-year-old boy needs about 3,000 calories a day (!), not far from the menu for the 220-pound "Man of Muscle."

Below I've presented a day's eating plan of 1,800 calories, perfect for kids between 4 and 6 years old. Adjust the serving sizes up or down for kids of different ages. I've chosen kid-friendly foods (like halibut, a fish without all the, well, *fishy* properties kids usually don't approve of. It's firm, white and somewhat "like chicken") and preparations (bread pudding they can make—kids like activity food). The earlier you introduce a wide range of foods, the better. They might not go for all of them—and I've learned you should never coax, bribe, threaten, force or punish a child about food issues—but the way to diversify their tastes is through regular exposure to all kinds of foods. You'll increase the odds of finding what they really like and allow them to develop an appreciation for more and more as time goes on.

My central piece of advice for getting healthy foods into kids and avoiding the not-so-healthy is no different than it is for grown-ups: Keep healthy snacks on hand at all times (fresh and dried fruit, nuts, granola mixes, yogurt, whole grain muffins) and don't stock what you don't want them to eat regularly (chips, ice cream, soda, commercial cookies . . .). Make treats *treats,* not a routine part of every day. Take a walk to the soft-serve cone shop or pick up a single-serve (1–2 oz) bag of chips for an afternoon hike.

BREAKFAST
2 oz (⅔ c) old-fashioned rolled oats
1 c water
1 (6 oz) cubed apple
1 tbsp dried cranberries
Pinch cinnamon
Microwave the oats 2 minutes and serve with:
4 oz (½ c) yogurt in bowl
1 tbsp honey (drizzle on)
4 oz (½ c) soy milk to drink

SNACK
3 oz (½ medium) banana
½ oz (1 tbsp) peanut butter

LUNCH
3 oz grilled chicken strips
2 oz (¾–1 c cooked) quinoa pasta with:
1 tbsp Parmesan
5 oz (¾–1 c) Braised Mixed Veggies*: green beans, scallion, carrot
    strips

SNACK

3 oz (½ c) berries

SUPPER

Celery sticks with:

Crema di Carciofi (Creamy Artichoke Dip)* and black olives

3 oz Halibut alla Pizzaiola (Halibut Pizza Style)* (simplify the
sauce to just tomatoes and parsley for sensitive taste buds, if
necessary)

8 oz (1 medium ear) corn on the cob *or* 2 oz (⅔ c cooked) Polenta*

DESSERT

Nicolletta (Hasty Bread Pudding)*

THE JOURNEY CONTINUES

The menu plans in this chapter give you a framework to work from
that the recipes in the next chapter will help you flesh out. I hope you
will enjoy your journey through the phases of The Diet Code, especially the ones that play out in the kitchen and at your table. Cracking
The Code will not only bring you to your ideal weight and provide
optimal health through excellent nourishment but will also free you
from the anxiety so much of us experience about food. Our bad
habits may be deeply ingrained, but the Italians know another way,
and there's no reason we can't adopt it as our own. So enjoy nature's
bounty, employ nature's proportions, and tune into the forgotten wisdom of our own bodies and those who have gone before us.

Pull your chair up to Leonardo's table.

CHAPTER TEN

The Diet Code Recipes

Those . . . who are inventors are interpreters of nature.
—LEONARDO DA VINCI

Any sufficiently advanced technology is indistinguishable from magic.
—ARTHUR C. CLARKE

Finally, it's time to *eat!* You've already learned how to put a basic Diet Code meal on the table—choose your Fundamental Foods, combine them in the proper proportion and prepare them simply. You could do very well in terms of nutrition, satisfaction and weight loss with no more than that, and you are more than welcome to do so. But the recipes I've created will make your life easier. They meet Diet Code requirements and are designed to get you to your ideal weight. Just as important to me is that they knock you out with how they look and taste. This is food meant to be *enjoyed*. It's also meant to be everyday food—meals you can realistically put on the table quickly after a long day; meals requiring no hard-to-find ingredients; meals most everyone (including kids) will like.

The dishes here are all specifically designed to work within The Diet Code, and some give you complete Diet Code proportions all in one meal. In most cases, I give you suggestions on what to serve with them to round out the meals appropriately. You've had glimpses of many of these dishes throughout this book and a preview of what these complete Diet Code meals look like in the previous chapter. Here's where you'll learn how easy it is to actually make them on your own.

You could certainly follow The Diet Code without ever using a Diet Code recipe. Once you look through these recipes, however, I don't think you'll want to.

—⚬—

My cooking has always been guided by the spirit of my Italian grandmother, Nona Louisa. She was of peasant stock herself, but her cooking was quite refined. Her food was rustic and simple, yet elegant. Not gourmet, but I've had meals at four-star restaurants that can't touch my grandmother's.

I remember the most basic things as the most extraordinary, like a salad of dandelion greens, onion, oil and vinegar, salt and pepper. Or her tomato sauce, composed merely of tomatoes, olive oil and garlic, but quite delicate, with an almost floral quality to it. She made her own pasta as well, manicotti so light it practically melted in your mouth and chewy ricotta-based dumplings called cavatelli.

Another simple dish with an ethereal quality was her shell peas (fresh from her garden) with bacon and minced onion bits sautéed so clear you could almost see through them, like glass. She made her own dried tomato paste; I remember watching her spread it on screens to dry in the sun. She had a woodstove in the basement, and each summer she fired it up for about a month straight to can and preserve much of the bounty of her garden. The aromas from her house were extraordinary, even when you were just walking by outside.

Every Friday at Sophia's, I'm very aware of the way my grandmother's spirit lives on. Friday is tomato soup day, and my customers go crazy over it. Every week someone raves about it and then asks me what's in it but never quite believes me when I tell them (crushed tomatoes, olive oil, mint and garlic). They'll ask, "But what makes it so glossy?" or, "But what makes it taste like flowers?" Or someone will ask about the soup of the day, pass when they hear it is tomato, and then come back to order some once they see (and smell) a bowl go by on its way to another table. When I coax that kind of complexity out of such basic things, I know my grandmother would approve and that my family heritage lives on.

The tastes, smells and sights of my grandmother's table still inspire all my culinary efforts. From my earliest childhood I have a distinct memory of how things *should* taste. Her food set the benchmark for me.

Of course, my grandmother could easily spend a whole day preparing one of her feasts. That may be a good fit with Mediterranean culture (from which we could learn much), but practically speaking, working in the kitchen for hours a day is simply not feasible or desirable for most Americans. What I've tried to do is recapture all that was wonderful about what she fed her family while adapting it to a modern pace of life. My goal is always *How close can I get to her standard . . . in half an hour?*

I aim for simple seasonal produce and employ traditional cooking techniques that enhance taste, aroma, texture and presentation, sidestepping the mire of trying to induce flavor by using a lot of ingredients or complicated procedures.

I never cooked with my grandmother, so I never learned her recipes directly. But I've been able to re-create their essence by using the Golden Proportion. A wide variety of my recipes will be included here, from that tomato soup to flourless chocolate cake and everything in between. As the single parent of three teenage children, I'm juggling the demands of running a business, raising children and nurturing my own creative talents. Therefore I have carefully honed these recipes to be nutritious, correctly proportioned, delightfully balanced in taste and texture—and also quick and easy to prepare. Most require a total of less than 30 minutes, and many take just 10 minutes, start to finish. There's even an entire five-course meal you can complete in an hour! This is food appealing and delicious enough for the most discriminating palates (both gourmet and juvenile). The emphasis is on fresh, wholesome, natural ingredients (available at most supermarkets), simply prepared. Excellent ingredients don't require much interference from you.

RECIPE TABLE OF CONTENTS

ANTIPASTI
Appetizers

ZUPPA e MINESTRE
Soups and Broths

CEREALI
Grains

INSALATA
Salad

VERDURE
Vegetables

PASTA

PESCE
Fish

UOVE
Eggs

POLLO
Chicken

CARNE
Meat

DOLCE
Dessert

FIVE-COURSE FEAST

RECIPE INDEX

—≈—

ANTIPASTI
Appetizers

—≈—

ZUPPA e MINESTRE
Soups and Broths

—◊—

CEREALI

Grains

—◊—

INSALATA
Salad

—ᴍ—

VERDURE
Vegetables

—ɱ—

PASTA

—ɱ—

PESCE
Fish

—ɱ—

UOVE

Eggs

—ↀ—

POLLO

Chicken

—ↀ—

CARNE

Meat

—ↀ—

DOLCE
Dessert

—∽—

FIVE-COURSE FEAST

ANTIPASTI / APPETIZERS

PUREA PUGLIESE   (Serves 4)
White Bean Spread

This spread is from eastern Italy. Serve it with bread, olives and a green salad or, more traditionally, Braised Greens (see recipe on p. 285).

- Puree in food processor or blender:
    19-oz can butter beans, cannellini beans or chickpeas, well drained
    2 tbsp fruity olive oil
    1 tbsp lemon juice
    1–2 cloves garlic or roasted garlic
    ½ tsp cracked black pepper
    Pinch sea salt, dried oregano or marjoram to taste

AGLIO ARROSTO
Roasted Garlic

Roasting considerably mellows garlic's usual pungency, so this creamy vegetable butter, loaded with minerals and antioxidants, makes a delicate spread for bread or vegetables or a subtly rich addition to other recipes. Serve it right from the oven as part of an antipasti array.

- Preheat oven to 425–450 degrees.
- Peel off the loose, outermost skin of:
    1 whole garlic bulb head
- Shear off tips (about top quarter of the bulb).

- Drizzle and sprinkle with:
  1 tsp olive oil
  Pinch sea salt
  Pinch rosemary or thyme
- Bake (forno) on a sheet pan or roasting dish for 20–30 minutes or until fragrant and soft.

CECI ALLA SARDEGNA
Sardinian Chickpea Salad

(Serves 8 to 10 as an appetizer or 4 as a main course)

These versatile chickpeas with fried sage and Arabic-influenced spices are equally tasty hot or cold (as an appetizer, with olives) or, as I serve it at Sophia's, as a bed for flaked white tuna. Tossed with pantacce pasta or wide spelt noodles, these ceci re-create what is one of the oldest pasta dishes in the world—akin to the *laganum* the Romans enjoyed based on a 3,000-year-old Greek preparation known as *laganon* (missing only the *garum*, or fermented fish sauce, so valued by the ancients).

- Drain and set aside:
  2 19-oz cans ceci (chickpeas)
- Sauté (saltere) in skillet over medium heat until fragrant:
  3 tbsp olive oil
  8 chopped fresh sage leaves
  2 cloves crushed garlic
  ¼ tsp sea salt
  ¼ tsp ground black pepper
  ¼ tsp thyme
  ⅛ tsp turmeric
  Pinch ground cinnamon to taste
- Add beans and toss to coat with oil.
- Remove from heat and moisten with:
  1 tbsp lemon juice (juice from ¼ lemon)

GAMBERI BRACE ALLA DIAVOLO   (Serves 4)
Grilled Devil's Shrimp

This is a great summer appetizer next to an icy Moretti beer, and it turns into a refreshing *secondo,* or main dish, when served atop a bed of long-grain rice smothered with a bright green sauté of snow peas, scallions and Italian or Thai basil.

- Marinate for 1 hour in plastic food-storage bag in refrigerator:
   1 lb cleaned raw jumbo shrimp with tails on
   ⅓ c Thai sweet chili sauce
   1 tbsp olive oil
   2 tsp sesame oil
   1 clove garlic, crushed
   ½ tsp dried basil or mint
   ½ tsp Thai hot chili sauce
- Preheat oven and grill pan to 550 degrees or heat outdoor grill.
- Thread shrimp onto four bamboo skewers.
- Grill (brace) 2 minutes each side to lightly char, or until shrimp are striped pink and black.
- Serve immediately.

CAPONATA   (Serves 4)
Sweet and Sour Eggplant

This Sicilian (Catanese) dish is usually served as a piquant appetizer but has found its way into Sophia's menu as a satisfying vegetarian sandwich, stuffed in a Tini roll (see recipe on p. 270) with a slice of provolone and served like a patty melt. Caponata is also perfection plated with a complementary lean protein in the form of its Sicilian sister, tuna. It's a revered combo at the bakery. At home I also like to serve it warm as an appetizer, with sardines or goat cheese and whole grain crackers.

This version of caponata is made, as befits a baker, in the oven rather than on the stove top. I add a few clean maple or cherry wood-chips to a separate small baking pan to impart an earthy smoked flavor, and those of you with a well-vented oven can do the same at home.

- Chop into 1-inch cubes:
  2 large eggplants
- Leave in a colander to drain for 1 hour after sprinkling with:
  1 tsp sea salt
- Preheat oven to broil; preheat grill pan and large ovenproof skillet.
- Chop into 1-inch pieces:
  1 large red bell pepper
  1 large green bell pepper
  2 stalks celery with leaves
- Toss peppers and celery with:
  1 tbsp olive or grapeseed oil
- Sear (salto) in grill pan, until tinged black. Then, remove from oven and set aside.
- Chop coarsely:
  3 large tomatoes
- Toss tomatoes with:
  2 tbsp turbinado sugar
  1 tbsp olive oil
  1 tbsp capers
- Sear (salto) tomatoes in skillet 3–4 minutes to tinge black, then remove from oven and set aside.
- Reduce oven to 475 degrees. Preheat baking sheet, and add wood-chips in a separate pan (if using).
- Toss eggplant with:
  3 medium onions, cubed
  1 tbsp olive oil
  ½ c crushed or chopped green or black olives
- Roast (arrosto) 30 minutes, turning once with a spatula after 15 minutes.

- Deglaze pan with:
  ¼ c red wine vinegar
- Add all the vegetables to the skillet, and reheat for 5 minutes.

CREMA DI CARCIOFI   (Serves 8)
Creamy Artichoke Dip

This is a delectable vegan mayo substitute. Spread it on slabs of beef-steak tomato or grilled tempeh, or use it as a dip for raw veggies. A 1-ounce (2-tablespoon) serving has only 50 calories and 3½ grams of fat.

- Drain:
  14-oz can artichoke hearts
- Puree in food processor with:
  2 tbsp fruity olive oil
  1 tsp lemon juice
  ¼ tsp sea salt

ZUPPA E MINESTRE / SOUPS AND BROTHS

UMBRIAN ACQUACOTTA (Serves 5)
Tomato Soup

This central Italian "cooked water" soup is simple and speedy to prepare. It is often served over a dense slab of semolina bread with a floating poached egg for a complete meal.

- In a saucepan, sauté over medium heat until just shy of golden:
  2–4 cloves garlic, slivered, in ¼ c olive oil
- Add:
  1½ tsp dried mint
  1–2 tbsp turbinado sugar
  3 c water
  2 28-oz containers crushed tomatoes
  2 packets (or 2 cubes or 2 tsp) high-quality chicken bouillon
- Bring to simmer (sobollire) over medium-high heat.
- Reduce to medium, and cook uncovered 5–10 minutes.
- Garnish with:
  Fresh-torn basil or parsley
  Cracked pepper

ACQUA FREDDA (Serves 4)
Italian Gazpacho

This refreshing "cold water" tomato soup is ultra-clean on the palate—no salt or oil. Quaff down endless amounts of it on a hot day when most food seems unappealing, but don't be surprised if you find yourself breaking off a bit of cheese and bread to go with it after all.

- Stir together in a 3- to 4-quart ceramic or plastic (not metal) container with lid:

  28-oz container crushed tomatoes

  28-oz container strained tomatoes

  ¾ c cold water

  ½ c lemon or lime juice

  3-oz can chopped green chilis

  ½ tsp red chili flakes

  ¼ c packed chopped parsley

- Cover and chill overnight to thoroughly cool the soup and set the flavors.

MINESTRA DI PESCE   (Serves 4)
Seafood Soup

This is a light, spicy and delectable summer soup made with fish and shrimp that's a snap to prepare in 15 to 20 minutes. And it's fat free. I keep this meal ultra-light by accompanying it only with an icy Peroni beer. Later in the evening, you can follow up with fruit and cheese.

- Bring to a boil in a stockpot:

  4 c water

  ¼ c anchovy (Thai) fish sauce

  1–2 tsp Thai chili garlic sauce

- Add:

  1 lb mixed cubed fish and shrimp

  6 oz (1 c) snow peas or filet beans (cut 2 inches long)

  2 small tomatoes, cut into wedges

  2–4 cloves garlic, slivered

- Simmer (sobollire) 6–10 minutes covered, then remove from heat.
- Add:

  2 scallions, sliced into 1-inch diagonals

  ½ c parsley or cilantro leaves

- Let stand 2 minutes.
- Serve garnished with a wedge of lime and chili flakes, if desired.

ZUPPA DI LENTICCE ALL 'ABRUZZESE (Serves 8–10)
Lentil Soup

This is a slow-simmered central Italian soup perfect for crisp autumn nights. Serve it with slices of a braised picnic shoulder ham.

- Sauté in a stockpot:
    2–4 cloves garlic, crushed
    ⅓ c olive oil
- Add:
    10 c (80 oz) water
    28-oz container crushed tomatoes
    1 lb dry green (or French indigo) lentils
    2 packets (or cubes) high-quality beef bouillon
    2 packets (or cubes) high-quality ham bouillon
    1 tsp dried basil
    1 tsp dried marjoram
    2 fresh bay leaves
- Bring to a boil over medium-high heat.
- Reduce to medium and cook, covered, for 1 hour to tenderize lentils.
- Add:
    2 lb carrots, peeled and cut into 1-inch diagonals
- Cook 20–30 minutes longer.

ROMAN FISH SOUP   (Serves 1)

This is a meal for one prepared in minutes that almost precisely represents phi in the relationship between macronutrients. Enjoy it with a glass of wine (5 ounces), which has been calorically figured into the meal, for a total of 499 calories. All together, that's 64 grams of carbohydrates, 27 grams of protein and 15 grams of fat. To get phi exactly would require 63.5 grams of carbohydrates, 24 grams of protein and 15 grams of fat. That's about as close as you're going to get in any recipe!

- Sauté (saltere):
  2 tsp olive oil
  1 oz (2 tbsp) sliced leeks
- Add and bring to a simmer:
  Pinch thyme
  ½ cube (½ tsp) chicken bouillon
  1 c water
- Add, then cover and poach for 5 minutes:
  1 c (8 oz) canned broad beans
  ½ c (1 oz) chopped kale
  3 oz salmon, cubed (fresh or vacuum packed)

PASSATA DI ZUCCA   (Serves 4)
Creamy Squash Soup

This is a velvety-rich northwestern Italian dish especially good served
with grilled sausage, leeks and mushrooms.

- Whisk together in a saucepan over medium heat:
  16 oz canned organic squash or pumpkin (or 2 c cooked pureed
      winter squash)
  1 fresh bay leaf
  2 c chicken stock (or 2 c water plus 1 cube or 1 tsp chicken
      boullion)
  1 tbsp butter
  1 tsp turbinado sugar
  ½ tsp lemon zest
  ½ tsp nutmeg
  ¼ tsp marjoram
  ¼ tsp ground white pepper
- Bring to a simmer. Cook 5 minutes, then remove from heat.
- Stir in:
  ¼ c cream

• Garnish with:
  Fresh sage leaf
  Pinch chili flakes or chili oil

CAVOLATA (Serves 4)
Cabbage and Pasta Soup

This is one of my favorite soups—both light and cheery and very fragrant, complex and filling. It's a meal in itself that will have almost anybody liking cabbage.

• Prepare al dente, according to package directions:
  4 oz (dry) baby shells or riccitelle pasta
• Drain and toss with a little olive oil. Set aside.
• In a 4-quart casserole, sauté over medium heat until golden:
  2 tbsp olive oil
  2 oz (4 strips) bacon, minced
  1 onion, diced
• Add and sauté until nearly translucent:
  2 medium potatoes, peeled and cut into ½-inch cubes
  1 carrot, peeled and cut into ½-inch cubes
• Add and bring to a boil over medium-high heat:
  4 c chicken broth (or 4 c water plus 2 cubes or 2 tsp chicken boullion)
  1 c (8 oz) small red beans
  4 bay leaves
  2 tsp dried mint
  ½ tsp thyme
• Add:
  12 oz cabbage (half of a 5- to 6-inch head) cut into ½- by 1-inch pieces
• Cook al dente, 15–20 minutes, then remove from heat.

- Add:
  Precooked pasta
  2 scallions, slivered into ⅛-inch-wide diagonals
- Serve garnished with:
  Parsley leaves
  Grated Parmesan or other hard Italian cheese

COMPAGNO DI SCUOLA   (Serves 1)
Tomato and Tuna Soup

This "school friend" soup, resurrected from my college days, is made almost entirely from canned goods from the pantry, delivering home-made comfort and high nutrition in five minutes. With either a beer or 2 ounces of whole grain crackers, this instant supper of about 550 calories has a nearly perfect Diet Code profile, with over 25 grams of protein.

- Measure into a microwave-safe dish with a cover:
  1 c packaged crushed tomatoes
  1 c canned cannellini or beans of choice, drained
  ½ c water
  2 oz (⅓ of a typical 6-oz can) tuna
  2 tsp olive oil
  1 bay leaf (optional)
  ½ tsp dried mint or basil
  Pinch sea salt
  1 clove garlic, crushed
- Cover and microwave 2½–3 minutes.
- Pour into bowl and sprinkle with:
  1 tbsp grated Parmesan or other hard Italian cheese
  Fresh parsley or basil (optional)

BRODO MISO (Serves 1)
Miso Broth

Though it makes an excellent aperitif for just about any meal, I have this in its most basic version first thing every morning. It makes up in seconds, easier even than a cup of tea or coffee. As long as you don't boil the soup itself (just the water, not the miso), this is an excellent way to reap the benefits of a fermented food like miso, with its probiotics and digestive enzymes. All for just 30 calories per serving, with 4 grams of carbs, 3 grams of protein and no fat.

Miso paste comes in a variety of flavors and textures, from light, golden, mild miso made from chickpeas or rice with young ferments to salty, dark, chestnut-brown brews of barley or soybeans aged up to three years. Traditionally, the Japanese choose their miso according to the season, consuming lighter ones in warmer weather. You can use whichever you like best, but you may find you naturally incline toward darker, heartier miso as it grows colder.

The Italians have almost as many terms for soup as the Inuit have for snow. *Brodo*—thin broth—evolved from the Old High German *brod,* table companion to *brot* (bread). And while miso isn't traditionally Italian, it is the most healthful broth you can drink short of laboriously authentic stock rendered from meat, bones or vegetables.

- In a teapot or saucepan, bring to a boil:
  1 c water
- Pour water into a teacup or small soup bowl and stir in:
  2 tsp miso paste
  1 tsp nori flakes with bonito and sesame seeds
- Add (optional):
  1 tbsp finely diced tofu
- Float on top your choice of:
  A few incredibly thin slices of mushroom
  Shaved scallions

CEREALI / GRAINS

POLENTA   (Serves 4–6)

Serve soft polenta just off the stove as a side dish or as a breakfast porridge with kefir (similar to yogurt) and honey. Or, follow the preparation below for versatile "hard" polenta to serve with Pesce al Cartoccio (see recipe on p. 300), Pollo alla Cacciatore (see recipe on p. 306), Halibut alla Pizzaiola (see recipe on p. 299) or alongside braised greens or asparagus.

- In a saucepan, stir together and bring to a simmer:
  - 1½ c (8 oz) **quick-cooking polenta (cornmeal)**
  - **6 c water**
  - **1 tsp sea salt**
- Cook, stirring often, at medium-low heat for 5 minutes or until thickened. Serve soft polenta immediately, if desired.
- To make hard polenta, spread in oiled pie plate or baking dish, press on plastic wrap to seal, and chill to set. Hard polenta can be re-heated quickly by microwaving it for 1 minute or browning it in a skillet with a little olive oil.

MEINI   (Serves 6)
Polenta (Cornmeal) Muffins

These golden polenta cornmeal "coins" from Lombardy are kin to corn muffins. Serve with comb honey or strawberry preserves in the morning; complement the corn protein with a cup of kefir or butter-milk for a real Old World taste sensation. They are also great eaten with grilled fish and vegetables on a summer evening.

- Preheat oven to 350 degrees.
- Whisk together and then set aside:
    8 oz (1½ c) polenta cornmeal
    1½ tsp baking powder
- Oil or butter a muffin-top mold pan.
- Beat together:
    1 egg
    ⅓ c milk or soy milk
    ⅓ c sunflower oil or light olive oil
    2 tbsp white wine (like pinot grigio)
    2 tbsp lemon juice
    3 tbsp honey
    ¼ tsp anise seed
    ¼ tsp dried rosemary
- Fold in polenta by hand until roughly mixed.
- Portion into molds (optional: sprinkle with demerara sugar crystals).
- Bake (forno) for about 20 minutes until golden on top with the rims just turning brown.

ALPINE BAKED PORRIDGE MUFFINS   (Serves 6)

These fragrant whole grain "muffins" are wheat-free, flourless and vegan, with no refined sugars. Day-old muffins can be reheated in a microwave for 30 to 60 seconds and crumbled into a bowl with milk or yogurt for a makeshift porridge—my oldest son's favorite.

- Line "Texas-size" muffin tins with paper liners and spray with food-release cooking spray.
- Preheat oven to 350 degrees.
- Toss together and set aside:
    6 oz (1⅔ c) oat flakes
    3 oz (¾ c) rye flakes
    3 oz (¾ c) spelt flakes

    2 tbsp flaxseeds

    2 tsp baking powder

    ½ tsp cinnamon

    ½ tsp coriander

    ½ tsp ginger

- Clean and cube, then set aside:

    1 large apple

- Beat together:

    ⅓ c light olive oil or sunflower oil

    ⅓ c maple syrup or Fruit Sweet fruit syrup

    1¾ c soy milk

    2 tbsp lemon juice

    1 tbsp vanilla

    ½ c raisins

- Mix grain mixture and apple into liquid. Let stand 2–3 minutes.
- Pour into muffin cups.
- Bake (forno) for 32–35 minutes.

TINI   (Makes 12 wedge-shaped rolls)

Rustic Rolls

I like to bake these homely but delicious rolls just long enough for them to show a little charring.

- In a 4-quart bowl, combine:

    18 oz (2⅛ c) water

    4 oz semolina

    20 oz unbleached bread flour

    ¼ c light olive oil

    2 tsp sea salt

    2 tbsp honey

    1 tbsp instant yeast

- Mix by hand until smooth.

- Let stand 30 minutes, then cover with plastic wrap and refrigerate overnight to develop flavor.
- Remove 2 hours before mealtime.
- Scrape dough out of bowl onto floured board, and divide into 3 pieces. Round each piece; rest on board under plastic for 1–1½ hours.
- Preheat oven to 500 degrees.
- Press and dimple out dough into three 10-inch disks.
- Quarter each circle into wedges, making 12 pieces.
- Slide onto preheated baking stone dusted with semolina or cornmeal.
- Bake (forno) 10–14 minutes, or until puffy and brown.

This ratio of water to flour, 18:24 or 3:4, also called *diatessaron,* is a Pythagorean standard hydration of 0.75 or 75% for many Italian breads (see appendix B).

QUINOA PORRIDGE   (Serves 4)

I can't say enough good things about this gluten-free, easy to digest, complete protein, ancient American grain. I love it as a breakfast cereal, and my preparation gives it a northern Italian, almost Eastern European, flavor. It also yields an almost perfect Diet Code profile, with 19 grams of protein and 400 calories per serving.

- In a saucepan over medium heat, lightly toast (3–5 minutes):
    8 oz (1⅓ c) Inca red quinoa (my favorite, an heirloom variety)
    2 tbsp poppy seeds
- Add and bring to a boil over medium-high heat:
    3 c water
- Cover, reduce heat to medium-low, and simmer (sobollire) for about 15 minutes, until water is absorbed. Add:
    4–6 chopped prunes or figs or 1½ oz (¼ c) other dried fruit
- Remove from heat and let stand, covered, about 10 minutes.
- Serve with:
    1 c buttermilk, kvass, yogurt or kefir
    Good honey to drizzle on top

CRESPELLE
(Serves 4; makes about 26 crepes)

Buckwheat Crepes

An ancient grain blend—buckwheat and spelt—from the Alpine reaches of Lombardy makes these healthy crepes a substantial and warming breakfast on a winter morning. Serve layered with sour cream or mascarpone and elderberry, plum or black raspberry preserves.

- Preheat a 6- to 8-inch nonstick skillet over medium heat.
- Whisk together in a 10-inch mixing bowl:
    4 eggs
    1½ c soy milk
    1 c water
    2 tbsp rum
    2 tbsp honey
    4 oz (1 c sifted) buckwheat flour
    4 oz (1 c sifted) whole spelt flour
    ½ tsp ground coriander or cardamom
- For each crepe: Drizzle hot skillet with:
    ¼ tsp sunflower oil
- Pour in 3 tbsp batter and swirl to evenly coat bottom of skillet.
- Cook each side 40–60 seconds until lightly flecked brown.
- Stack and serve immediately in piles of 6 crepes.

PANISSA
(Serves 4)

Bread Pilaf

Serve this "little bread" pilaf—something like American stuffing or dressing—alongside hard-boiled eggs and grilled zucchini or broiled pollock and filet beans accented with a pinch of caraway seed.

This dish works only with a bread that will create a texture and have a color like bulgur wheat (of tabouli salad fame), so choose dark, whole meal or seeded breads like the Bavarian imports, and leave the white and even, dense amber sourdoughs for conventional stuffings or bread pudding.

- Preheat oven to 325 degrees.
- Crumble until pea-sized and spread on a baking sheet in one thin, even layer:
    8 oz (1½ c) whole meal bread
- Toast 15–20 minutes, turning over with a spatula halfway through, and set aside.
- In a skillet over medium heat, sauté until golden:
    1 tbsp olive oil
    1 small onion, minced
- Remove from heat and fold in bread.
- In saucepan over medium-high heat, bring to a simmer:
    ½ c chicken stock (or ½ c water plus ¼ cube or ¼ tsp chicken bouillon)
- Drizzle broth over bread and toss to moisten. Add (if desired):
    Chopped parsley to taste
- Serve immediately.

PHI BREAD   (Makes a 3-pound loaf)

This is my original Fibonacci loaf recipe from almost two decades ago. This bread, linking 3,000 years of human history, is built on a Genesis-like outline of seven days of creation. Just try to wait and eat it until the seventh day of rest!

The dough ferments without refrigeration, so it is best made when ambient room temperature is between 70 and 80 degrees. The finished product will keep for five days in a bread box or waxed paper bag—it's what my friend the food critic John Thorne would call "the durable loaf," designed to age like wine or cheese, command respect and deliver real sustenance.

The standard recipe follows, but first check out this chart below, which shows off the use of the Fibonacci sequence (1, 1, 2, 3, 5, 8, 13,

21, 34, 55, 89 . . .). (It may not be obvious from the recipe, but even the amount of salt reflects phi: Multiplying the total amount of flour (32 ounces) times 0.01618 gives you 0.52 ounces, or 2½ teaspoons (1 teaspoon of salt is approximately 0.21 ounces).

Day	Water (ounces)	Flour (ounces)	Weight of additions (ounces)
1	1	1	2
2	Add 1	plus 2	3
3	Add 2	plus 3	5
4	Add 3	plus 5	8
5	Add 5	plus 8	13
6	Add 8	plus 13	21

- To make the sourdough sponge starter, in a 10- to 12-inch ceramic or plastic bowl with a fitted lid, mix:
  - **1 oz (1 tbsp) cool water**
  - **1 oz organic whole wheat, rye or spelt flour**
- Cover and let stand overnight.
- The next day, add to the bubbly sponge formed by natural yeasts:
  - **1 oz (1 tbsp) cool water**
  - **2 oz organic unbleached or partially sifted wheat flour**
- Cover to keep dough from skinning over and drying out, and let stand overnight again.
- On day three, mix in:
  - **2 oz (2 tbsp) cool water**
  - **3 oz organic sifted wheat flour**
- Cover and let stand another night.
- On the following day, mix in:
  - **3 oz (3 tbsp) cool water**
  - **5 oz organic sifted wheat flour**
- Cover and let stand overnight.
- Then add:
  - **5 oz (5 tbsp) cool water**
  - **8 oz organic sifted wheat flour**
- Cover and let stand one more night.
- On the sixth day (bake day!) of the process, add:

8 oz (1 c) cool water

13 oz organic sifted wheat flour

2½ tsp sea salt

- Knead for 1 minute, then rest dough in covered bowl for *21* minutes.
- Knead dough again briefly (1 minute); cover and rest *34* minutes.
- Scrape out of bowl onto a lightly floured surface, round into a ball, cover with a sheet of plastic wrap or a cotton cloth, and let rest *55* minutes.
- Gather up and re-round loaf. Place seam side–up into a bowl lined with a clean cloth dusted with flour. Cover with cloth and let rest *89* minutes (1½ hours).
- Meanwhile, preheat oven to 400 degrees, with a pizza stone or heavy baking sheet on the middle rack. (Using a pizza stone is definitely preferable; it gives the bread more spring and better crust development.)
- Flip the loaf from the bowl onto a wooden peel or a thin, wide board dusted with bran or cornmeal. Cut a cross into the top of the loaf. Slide off the peel onto the pizza stone or baking sheet in the oven.
- Bake (forno) *55* minutes to a dark caramel color.

BAKER'S LUNCH

(Serves 1)

This is a favorite meal of Italian stonecutters, including Michelangelo, Leonardo's archrival, and it comes as close to reproducing phi exactly as you're ever going to get. With 372 calories, the Baker's Lunch has 47 grams of carbs, 19 grams of protein and 12 grams of fat—where phi would be precisely 50.83 grams of carbs, 19.42 grams of protein and 12 grams of fat.

Serve it with a nutrient-dense Italian slaw or tomato and basil salad.

- Assemble on a plate:

    3-oz slab artisanal sourdough bread, like Phi Bread (see recipe on p. 273), or whole grain peasant bread

    1 oz aged Asiago cheese

    ½ oz (6 fillets) white anchovy

BISTECA DI PANE

(Serves 4)

Bread Steak

A Tuscan would call it *fettunta,* or you might think of it as bruschetta. The Catalans of Spain revere this as *pa amb tomaquet;* elsewhere Spaniards call it *sopa seca,* or "dry soup." But this more ancient version, literally "steak of bread," is simple grilled bread. It's named for the way it's eaten off the plate with a knife and fork, like a piece of meat. Sometimes I serve it American style, alongside bacon and eggs, perhaps with a side of grilled tomatoes with olive oil and oregano. The more traditional presentation would have it laid down like a plate and piled high with food (perhaps Braised Greens [see recipe on p. 285] or a fried egg) to soak up its juices before being the last thing eaten.

- Preheat oven and grill pan to 500 degrees. (Alternatively, you can prepare this on the stove top over medium-high heat.)
- Select:
  4 1-inch-thick slices of dense, chewy sourdough peasant bread, like Phi Bread (see recipe on p. 273)
- Drizzle or brush with:
  4 tsp olive oil (½ tsp for each side of each slice)
- Place bread in grill pan and toast until lightly browned, with sear marks.
- Rub each slice with either or both:
  1 clove garlic, peeled
  ½ ripe tomato
- Sprinkle to taste with:
  Sea salt
  Fresh-ground black pepper

PANZANELLA

(Serves 4)

Bread Salad

Modern versions of this recipe tend to be jazzed up quite a bit—
"more suitable for the appetite of the clerk than the peasant" as my
old friend and patron, food critic John Thorne, put it. So my panzanella doesn't have cheese or roast peppers or even tomatoes, aiming to get closer to the peasant bread and herb dish of Leonardo's day.
Serve with plain cold roast chicken, and perhaps chilled cantaloupe
for dessert.

- Tear or cut into 1-inch cubes:
  - **8 oz (2 c) dense peasant bread**
- Toss in a bowl and sprinkle, to moisten, with:
  - **¼ c water**
- In a separate bowl, toss together:
  - **1 small (6-inch) cucumber, peeled, seeded and cubed**
  - **2 scallions, split lengthwise and cut into 2-inch lengths**
  - **¼ c packed torn basil leaves**
  - **2 oz or 1 c loose small arugula or baby dandelion leaves**
  - **1 tsp fresh oregano leaves**
- For dressing, combine and toss into greens:
  - **3 tbsp peppery olive oil**
  - **1–2 tbsp red wine vinegar (to taste)**
- Fold in bread, and then sprinkle on:
  - **1 tsp cracked black pepper**
  - **½ tsp coarse sea salt**

INSALATA / SALAD

INSALATA DI CAVOLO   (Serves 4–6)
Cabbage Salad

The premier salad at Sophia's is this very light and nutritious coleslaw. It will last up to four days refrigerated (without dressing), so one slaw session can go far. The Lemon Caper Dressing is very good on many vegetables, including asparagus, avocados, tomatoes and mushrooms.

- Prepare Lemon Caper Dressing, combining ingredients below and letting stand for 30 minutes:
    ¼ c lemon or lime juice
    1 tsp lemon or lime zest (optional)
    2–4 tbsp fruity olive oil
    1 tbsp capers
    1 tsp turbinado sugar or honey
- Meanwhile, toss in a large serving bowl:
    1 lb green cabbage (half of a medium-size, 6-inch head), cleaned, cored and shredded into strips about ⅛ inch wide
    4 oz white or red onion (1 medium [2½-inch] bulb) or scallions, slivered
    ½ c (1½ oz) Italian parsley leaves
    ½ tsp aniseed
    ½ tsp dried mint
    ½ tsp chili flakes
- Stir dressing and spoon over slaw just before serving, seasoning to taste with:
    Sea salt

INSALATA ALLA NAPOLETANA (Serves 6)

Neapolitan Cauliflower Salad

Visually stunning and varied in taste and textures, this is a truly great summer salad served alongside crusty bread and grilled fish or skewered lamb.

- Cut into 1- to 1½-inch florets:
  1 head cauliflower
- Steam or blanch until just tender; you should be able to pierce it with a knife tip.
- Rinse immediately under cool water in colander; drain or pat dry.
- Toss with:
  4 cloves garlic, crushed
  2 tbsp capers
  6 anchovies, chopped
  3 Italian vinegar-pickled sweet red peppers, sliced
  1 c parsley leaves (3 oz)
  1 small can black olives, drained (or ½ c pitted olives of your choice)
- Dress with:
  ¼ c rice or white balsamic vinegar
  3 tbsp fruity olive oil
  ½ tsp red chili flakes
  Sea salt to taste
- Let stand in refrigerator for 30 minutes before serving to allow flavors to meld.

CAESAR SALAD SOPHIA   (Serves 6)
Caesar Salad for the Wise

The great Caesar salad, a New World invention with an assumed Italian heritage, is a classic no matter its lineage. My twist is to create an authentic whole-egg dressing that is cooked for safety, like the very authentic custard zabaglione. This recipe yields 1 cup of dressing, enough for twelve. Perhaps you want to make the grilled version later on in the week, or try using the other ½ cup for a batch of egg salad in place of mayonnaise. The dressing keeps for about a week in the refrigerator.

- Whisk in a saucepan:
  - **1 egg**
  - **⅓ c olive oil**
  - **2 tbsp white balsamic vinegar**
  - **1½ tsp anchovy paste**
- Heat (sbollentare) while whisking over medium-low heat until creamy. Do not boil.
- Remove from heat, and then whisk in:
  - **3–4 tbsp lemon juice**
  - **1 tbsp crushed garlic**
  - **1 tsp Worcestershire sauce**
  - **1 tsp Dijon mustard**
- Toss this dressing with:
  - **2 lb torn romaine or Boston lettuce**
  - **¼ c grated Romano**
  - **Cracked black pepper to taste**
- Top with:
  - **Freshly shaved Parmesan to taste**

VARIATION: GRILLED CAESAR SALAD   (Serves 4)

- Preheat oven and grill pan to 500 degrees.
- Cut lengthwise into halves:
  1 head romaine lettuce
- Cut into 4 long wedges, and place in the grill pan.
- Grill romaine 2–3 minutes on each side to get sear marks.
- Place one quarter onto each serving plate, and top with:
  2 tbsp dressing
  Freshly shaved Parmesan to taste

MISTICANZA   (Serves 4)
Wild Greens Salad

In 1614, Renaissance "foodie" and socialite Giacomo Castelvetro, sequestered in England to escape the Inquisition, came face to face with another horror: the British proclivity for lots of meat and pastry. So he wrote and distributed a book, *The Fruit, Herbs and Vegetables of Italy*, in hopes of rescuing his rescuers from an inner torment of indigestion, impacted intestines, flatulence and obesity. His dream? To teach the Brits how to make a salad. Almost four centuries later, our own once-British country still struggles.

Candidates for Castelvetro's salad included chicory, cabbage, cress, endive, lettuce hearts, cucumber, purslane, valeriana, basil, mint, fennel, sorrel, lemon balm, salad burnet, tarragon, rocket (arugula), borage, rosemary—and violets. Experiment with all these and more. Try some things you've always bypassed at the grocery store. And please: Forget the iceberg (essentially a nutritional zero). Make Castelvetro happy and make a real salad.

• Select 1¼ lb of mixed greens, using the following as a suggestion only:

    8 oz (3 c) radicchio

    8 oz (3 c) frisée endive

    3 oz (1½ c) arugula (rocket)

    ½ oz (½ c) basil leaves, torn

    ½ oz (⅓ c) chives, chopped into spiky 1½-inch lengths

• Wash leaves by plunging into water; then shake and gently towel dry (Castelvetro's method) or dry in a salad spinner (mine).

• Tear or cut the leaves into 2-inch pieces.

• In a large bowl, toss the greens with the chives.

• Dress with good oil, vinegar and sea salt, or try one of the dressings that follow.

GETTING DRESSED

Castelvetro didn't stop at just identifying greens when instructing the British on vegetables—naturally he advised them on dressing them as well. He counseled, "Never do as the . . . uncouth nations do—pile the badly washed leaves, neither shaken nor drained, up in a mound . . . then throw on a little salt, not much oil and far too much vinegar without even stirring. And all this done to produce a decorative effect, where we Italians would much rather feast the palate than the eye."

He goes on to reveal, "The secret of a good salad is *plenty of salt, generous oil and little vinegar* [italics added], hence the text of the Sacred Law of Salads, *Insalata ben salata poco aceto e ben oliata.*"

WARM ORANGE DRESSING (Serves 4)

Wilder greens are slightly bitter (making them very beneficial for digestion), so they mate nicely with a sweet dressing. Try this one with radicchio, endive and arugula.

- Whisk together and heat in a small skillet on medium heat until just warmed:
  - **2 tbsp olive oil**
  - **1 tbsp white balsamic vinegar**
  - **1 tbsp orange juice**
  - **1 tbsp orange honey**
  - **¼ tsp crushed fennel seed**
- Drizzle right away over greens and garnish with:
  - **Pine nuts or**
  - **Shaved Paremsan**

BALSAMIC VINAIGRETTE (Serves 4)

This dressing is great for tomatoes, scallions and onions, and for grilled mushrooms, beets or peppers—all complemented with shaved Parmesan.

- Whisk together:
  - **3 tbsp olive oil**
  - **1 tbsp high-quality aged balsamic vinegar**
  - **1 tsp crushed garlic (optional)**
  - **¼ tsp toasted anise, cumin or caraway seeds (optional)**

WALNUT WHITE WINE DRESSING   (Serves 4)

I like to use this to make blanched green beans, grilled celery or baby spinach more exotic. Garnish with crushed walnuts or a crumbled blue-veined cheese.

• Whisk together:
  2 tbsp walnut oil
  1 tbsp white wine
  1 tbsp rice vinegar or white balsamic vinegar
  ⅛ tsp ground fenugreek
  ½ tsp turbinado sugar
  ½ tsp fresh thyme leaves
  Sea salt to taste

VERDURE / VEGETABLES

Here I eliminate the fear factors that keep people from venturing into a greater variety of vegetables—*I don't know what to do with them, and even if I did, it would take too long anyway*—and focus on getting a dozen of the most nutritionally dense vegetables available onto your table regularly. (With The Diet Code, you will effortlessly meet the new 2005 government recommendations for nine servings of fruits and vegetables [4½ cups] a day.) These, like all the Fundamental Foods called for, are not pricey gourmet items but are available in most any supermarket—and were available to Leonardo as well. They are also the most metabolically potent foods available—literally life savers.

ERBAZZONE ALLA BRASATA (Serves 6)
Braised Greens

Braising is *the* technique for cooking leafy greens, whether cabbage, kale, collards or chard, and it works as well for other green veggies like broccolini, asparagus and filet beans (fine, thin green beans).

Serve braised greens with warm Polenta (see recipe on p. 268) or Borlotti alla Boscaiolo (see recipe on p. 292), plus fried eggs, grilled sausage, fish or tempeh. Then voilà! You've got one of my Five Fundamental Meals.

Cleaning *and* cooking greens for six people will take about 15 minutes altogether. If you don't have that kind of time, try pre-prepping greens as I do at Sophia's, tossing a single-serving amount of greens with seasonings into a plastic food-storage bag (but without sea salt). They'll keep that way for up to a week in the refrigerator. Then, when you're hungry for greens, just pull out a bag, and you're ready in just a few minutes.

If that's still not fast enough for you, you can shave some time off by microwaving the greens and seasonings in a 9-inch round, hard plastic microwave-safe container with a loose lid—about 2 minutes for a single serving of chard, and about 4 minutes for kale.

- Plunge wash (in a sink or a bucket of water), then shake dry lightly (you want to retain some water for braising):
  24–30 oz (9–10 c) leafy greens
  6 oz (¾ c) leeks
- Remove from the greens any stems or ribs wider than half the thickness of a pencil, then slice about ⅜ inch wide (up to 1 inch for softer chard and choi).
- Chop leeks into 1-inch lengths.
- Preheat a large wok or skillet over medium heat, then add greens, leeks and:
  ¼ c olive oil
  2–4 tbsp water
  3–4 cloves garlic, slivered or crushed
- Braise, tossing with tongs to cook evenly, for about 4–6 minutes, or until just tender and still bright (do not singe brown), with little or no accumulated water in the pan bottom. Cover pan if necessary to keep moist, or remove lid to allow evaporation.
- Add to taste:
  Sea salt
  Fresh-ground pepper

VARIATION 1: GREENS FOR MEAT LOVERS (Serves 6)

Just a small amount of pancetta or bacon makes an amazing flavor contribution without adding much fat (a strip of bacon has less fat than 2 teaspoons of olive oil). Here's how you make it fresh. I keep some precooked diced bacon or ham in the fridge, so it's quick to toss into greens.

• Sauté (saltere) in pan before adding greens:

   6 strips of bacon or 3 oz (scant ½ c) pancetta affunicata (fatty "Italian bacon"), minced
• Finish as above, omitting olive oil.

VARIATION 2: MICRO MEAL (Serves 1)

Thanks to the microwave, this is a near-instant version of one of my Five Fundamental Meals. Serve with a 1-ounce hunk of cheese or grated Parmesan.

• Place in a hard plastic microwave-safe container with loose lid:

   6 oz (¾ c) hard Polenta (see recipe on p. 268)
• Cover with:

   4–5 oz (1½ c) greens, cleaned and chopped

   1 oz (2 tbsp) leeks, cleaned and chopped

   ½ clove garlic, crushed (½ tsp)

   2 tsp olive oil

   1 tsp water

   1 tbsp precooked bacon (optional)
• Crack into nest of raw greens:

   1–2 eggs
• Cover dish and microwave 4–5 minutes until greens are tender and eggs are done to your liking.
• Add to taste:

   Sea salt

   Fresh-ground black pepper

BRAISED GREEN VEGETABLES   (Serves 6)

- Rinse:

   **24 oz (8 c) broccolini, raab, or asparagus, cut into 5-inch
   lengths, or snow peas or filet beans**

   **6 oz (¾ c) leeks, scallions or green onions, split lengthwise and
   cut into 1-inch lengths**

- Microwave the just-washed veggies (with water still clinging to
  them), covered, for 1 minute to blanch (optional). This helps the
  braising occur more evenly and effortlessly.
- Preheat a large wok or skillet over medium heat. Then add veggies
  and:

   ¼ c olive oil

   2–4 tbsp water

   3–4 cloves garlic, slivered

   Pinch rosemary, oregano, thyme or other herb

- Braise, tossing with tongs to cook evenly, for about 4–6 minutes, or
  until just tender and still bright (do not singe brown), with little or
  no accumulated water in the pan bottom. Cover pan if necessary to
  keep moist, or remove lid to allow evaporation.
- Add to taste:

   Sea salt

   Fresh-ground pepper or chili flakes

- Serve with:

   Lemon or lime wedges

ASPARAGI GRIGLIATA   (Serves 4)

Grilled Asparagus

I grill (brace) *something* probably five times a week; this particular
recipe says "asparagus," but you can also use it for baby bok choi,
halved (lengthwise) zucchini, leeks, tomatoes, onions, radicchio and
more. Grilled veggies go well with boiled grains, like couscous, and
baked or roasted fish or meat. (Varying the cooking techniques ap-

plied at any given meal keeps interest and appreciation high; for this same reason, grilled meats are nice with braised vegetables and baked potatoes.)

As for the asparagus, I personally love it with a sprinkle of nori/bonito/sesame seed condiment from an Asian food store, featuring smoky shaved tuna and toasted seaweed (in which case you might want to omit the oregano). Or, take a more Italian approach if you like: Dress it with a few drops of white truffle oil.

- Prepare grill or preheat oven and grill pan to 550 degrees.
- Snap or cut into 5-inch lengths:
  1½ lb asparagus
- Toss in a bowl or plastic food-storage bag with:
  2–3 tbsp grapeseed oil
  1 tsp oregano
  ½ tsp sea salt
- If you're cooking out, arrange asparagus in a single layer in a grill basket and secure by locking handle.
- Indoors, arrange one layer deep in grill pan.
- Sear (salto) 2–3 minutes each side (outdoors or in) to tinge black.
- Serve immediately with:
  Shaved Parmesan
  Lemon wedges

ZUCCHINI AL FORNO   (Serves 6)

Oven-Roasted Zucchini

Juniper marinade makes this baker's preparation of summer squash intriguing. Serve warm over white beans or cold with pasta and grilled chicken.

- Mix dressing and let stand:
  2 tbsp fruity olive oil
  2 tbsp sherry or marsala

¼ c rice vinegar

1 tbsp turbinado sugar

½ tsp chili flakes

16–20 juniper berries, crushed with the back of a spoon, rolling pin, or mortar and pestle. (Look for these little purple-blue seedpods in jars in the spice section of your health food store or supermarket. These waxy berries are common in Italian cooking, used mostly with game.)

• Preheat oven to broil.
• Split lengthwise and cut into 2- to 3-inch sections:
  6 small zucchini
• Peel and cut into ½-inch wedges:
  2–3 medium onions
• Chunk into 6–8 pieces each:
  3 bell peppers—1 each, red, orange and yellow
• Brush clean and halve:
  11-oz package "baby bella" mushrooms
• Toss vegetables with:
  2 tbsp sunflower oil
  1 tsp sea salt
  1 tsp thyme
  2 cloves garlic, crushed
• Broil on baking sheet 5–6 minutes to just singe, then turn oven to 500 degrees and roast (arrosto) 5–6 minutes longer.
• Cool slightly, then toss with dressing.

POTATE AL RAMERINO   (Serves 4)
Rosemary Roast Potatoes

This is a standard in almost any Italian cookbook, and it couldn't be simpler: Cube potatoes, toss with herbs and oil, and roast at 400 degrees for 40 minutes. My twist is a strategy that cuts the usual cooking time in thirds. The ingredients (all except sea salt) can be microwaved and tossed together as much as four days in advance, then stored in plastic food-storage bags in the refrigerator. Divide into serving-size bags if you don't plan on roasting them all at once. For a change of pace, try swapping out the rosemary in favor of sage.

- Wash, and pierce each once or twice with a knife:
  2 lb Yukon Gold potatoes
- Microwave for about 8 minutes until knife tender.
- Cool and cut into 1-inch cubes.
- Toss potatoes with:
  4 oz (¾ c) chopped onion
  4 rosemary sprigs
  ¼ c light olive oil
  1 tsp fresh-ground black pepper
- To finish cooking, preheat oven and large skillet to 475 degrees.
- Roast (arrosto) potatoes 10–12 minutes until nicely browned. Turn once or twice with tongs or spatula, adding a bit more oil if necessary to keep from sticking.
- Add:
  Sea salt to taste

ROASTED ORANGE WINTER VEGETABLES

(Serves 4)

This works just as well with winter squash and can be prepared ahead.

- Cut in half crosswise and stand on microwavable plate cut side-down:
  2 lb (4 medium) sweet potatoes or 6- to 7-inch buttercup or other winter squash, scooped out and peeled
- Microwave 8 minutes for sweet potato or 10–12 minutes for squash, until knife tender.
- Cool and cut into 1-inch cubes.

- Toss sweet potatoes or squash with:

  4 oz (¾ c) onion, chopped

  2 apples, cubed

  ¼ c sunflower oil or light olive oil

  8 sage leaves, scissored into thin strips

  1 tsp fresh-ground pepper

  1 tsp coriander, nutmeg, aniseed or caraway
- To finish cooking, preheat oven and large skillet to 475 degrees.
- Roast (arrosto) sweet potatoes 10–12 minutes or until nicely browned. Turn once or twice with tongs or spatula, adding a bit more oil if necessary to keep from sticking.
- Add:

  Sea salt to taste

BORLOTTI ALLA BOSCAIOLO   (Serves 4–6)
Rustic Chili

While I built my own log home, these "woodcutter's style" beans were a welcome dish after a day spent swinging an axe. Fortified with potassium-rich molasses, this is an instant hit as a twist on vegetarian chili or accompanied by a few slices of imported hard salami for a protein boost.

- Sauté (saltere) in a 12-inch skillet over medium-low heat until fragrant:

  ¼ c olive oil

  2 cloves garlic, crushed

  2 bay leaves
- Add:

  28-oz container crushed tomatoes

  2 19-oz cans borlotti, kidney or cranberry beans, drained

  1–2 tbsp molasses

  ½ tsp rosemary

½ **tsp sea salt**
½ **tsp ground black pepper**
- Bring to a simmer over medium-high heat.
- Reduce heat to medium-low and cook, uncovered, to desired consistency, 10–20 minutes.
- Let stand 5 minutes before serving.

TEMPEH WITH ONIONS (Serves 2)

Tempeh is an Indonesian sprouted soybean cake often blended with sprouted grains like rice, millet or barley. It's a vegan dream food, affording as much protein per ounce as lamb or eggs (4.5 grams). It also has a significant amount of carbohydrate (12 grams per 4-ounce serving) and fat (8 grams per 4-ounce serving), so a strict Diet Code dinner would pair it with a starchy vegetable like butternut squash (or a premium 12-ounce beer!) instead of a full serving of bread, rice or pasta. Or, smother it in onions, as below; 6 ounces of onion provide another 12 grams of carbs for a near-perfect Diet Code profile, with a good 20 grams of protein and about 415 calories. It makes a refreshingly light breakfast with a frosty glass of fresh-squeezed orange juice (8 ounces).

- Slice crosswise into ¾-inch by 3-inch strips:
  8-oz package tempeh
- Slice lengthwise into ½-inch wedges:
  2 medium (12 oz) onions
- Toss onions and tempeh gently in bowl with:
  1 tbsp sunflower oil or grapeseed oil
  ¼ **tsp sea salt**
  ¼ **tsp caraway seed**
  ¼ **tsp marjoram**
- Preheat large skillet on medium heat. Add tempeh-onion mixture, and sauté (saltere) until golden, about 6–8 minutes.

GRILLED TEMPEH   (Serves 6)

Like eggplant, tempeh can absorb a lot of oil, and many recipes are prone to indulging it. Grilling avoids that trap. This super-simple preparation is one of my favorites. It goes best with softer, juicier foods like mashed potatoes or winter squash; sauerkraut, braised spinach or chard; or leeks sautéed with mushrooms and basil. Or, serve as an open-faced sandwich with Bavarian-style bread, slivered red onion, beefsteak tomato and Crema di Carciofi (see recipe on p. 260). This recipe is for six servings, because once you've got the grill pan going, fill it up knowing that tempeh keeps very well in the fridge (up to a week). Just reheat it in the microwave for 1 minute.

- Preheat oven and grill pan to 550 degrees.
- Cut in half, for a total of 6 pieces about 3½ inches square:
  3 8-oz packages tempeh
- Marinate in:
  ⅓–½ c favorite Asian grilling sauce or BBQ sauce
  1 tbsp grapeseed oil
- Grill (brace) 3 minutes on each side to get black sear marks.

PASTA

SUGO AL POMODORO (Serves 6)
Simplest Tomato Sauce

This is the essential red sauce of five irreducible components. You can dress it up with herbs, although to my taste, anything more than fresh-torn basil leads to confusion.

- In a saucepan or skillet over medium-low heat, sauté:
   3–4 cloves garlic, slivered
   ⅓ c fruity olive oil
- Cook the garlic until translucent but not colored. Then add:
   2 28-oz containers crushed tomatoes
   2 tbsp turbinado sugar (necessary to mollify the acidity of the tomatoes)
   ¼ tsp sea salt
- Bring to a simmer and cook for 10–30 minutes on low heat, depending on the consistency you want.

   This sauce may be made well ahead of time and refrigerated for up to a week. Allow an average of ¾–1 cup sugo per person.

CAVATELLI (Serves 4–6)
Pasta Dumplings

I have fond memories of making my Nona Louisa's Neapolitan version of the better-known northern Italian gnocchi with my daughter when she was only about three years old—and too short to work the dough at the table, so I laid a sheet of plastic on the floor so we could kneel there to shape the cavatelli. They are still her favorite!

Serve 1 cup per person with ¾–1 cup Sugo al Pomodoro (see recipe on p. 295). Add 3–5 ounces grilled sausage or chicken and garnish with fresh-torn basil leaves and a bit of grated Parmesan for a fully balanced meal.

- In a mixing bowl, combine:
  1 egg, beaten with ½ tsp sea salt
  1 lb ricotta
  6 oz (1½ c) spelt or unbleached wheat flour
- Knead smooth with spatula; cover and chill ½ hour.
- Pinch off ½-cup–size balls.
- Hand roll (on lightly floured surface) into finger-thick ropes.
- Cut 1-inch segments; drag and roll with the back tines of a fork to curl each little "plug" into fat crescents.
- Bring 1 gallon of salted water to boil in a stockpot and poach cavatelli, a dozen at a time, until they float.
- Remove with strainer to plate. Drizzle with olive oil to keep from sticking.

TRECCHE ALLE SARDE   (Serves 2)
Pasta with Sardines

This authentic Venetian dish makes a light but satisfying meal *in less than 15 minutes*. Accompany it with a salad of mixed greens and an icy beer or chilled white wine, like an Orvieto.

- Bring 1 quart of water to a boil in a saucepan. Cook 4–6 oz trecche or gemelli pasta al dente, according to package instructions. (This recipe lends itself well to whole grain spelt and kamut pasta in those shapes.)
- Meanwhile, in a skillet, "melt" or sauté over low heat:
  4-oz can brisling (tiny) sardines in their oil
  2–3 tbsp olive oil
  2 cloves garlic, slivered

- Gently mash sardines to nearly a paste, heating gently to just warm through. (No added salt is necessary because of the sodium content of the canned fish.)
- Drain and toss in pasta.
- Transfer to plates and garnish liberally with:
  Minced Italian parsley leaves
  Cracked pepper
  Lemon wedges
  Grated Parmesan or similar hard cheese

PUTTANESCA (Serves 4)
Pasta and Salmon with Puttanesca Sauce

This is a bit of a stretch from the original slap-dash "naughty girl's" pasta and requires a little more fuss (juggling four pots and pans) than does my usual fare. But it is so striking and so *very* tasty that it's worth it. This is not the time to go all out for a dessert, too, but it *is* the perfect time for coffee gelato from a freezer container.

I like a wide noodle for this dish, like pappardelle or spinach fettuccine or, for the daring, tonnarelli al nero—flat black pasta made with squid ink, which *looks* incredible. It won't be as elegant, but you can simplify this dish a bit by using a drained can of white tuna or vacuum-packed salmon instead of the poached fresh fish.

- Bring 1 gallon of salted water (for the pasta) to a boil in a stockpot on high heat. Use a back burner; you're going to be busy with the front ones!
- Put a saucepan with 2 inches of water (for poaching the fish) over medium heat on your other back burner.
- Combine in a small saucepan and set aside:
  ½ c cream
  1 tsp anchovy paste
  2 oz (¼ c) Fontina, cut into ½-inch cubes

- Cut in quarters and set aside:

  12 oz salmon fillet
- Coarsely chop and set aside in a bowl:

  2 medium onions

  2 medium tomatoes

  ½ c whole or sliced olives—choose black or green to offset the color of the pasta

  1 tbsp capers
- When you are ready to begin cooking—dinner can be ready in about 10 minutes at this point—and the pasta water is at a rolling boil, add and cook according to package directions:

  8 oz (½ of a 1-lb package) dry pasta
- Meanwhile, heat a large skillet on medium-high heat and sear (salto) veggies, using tongs to turn, in:

  ¼ c olive oil
- The poaching saucepan should be showing "champagne bubbles" (on medium heat). Gently lower the salmon pieces into the hot bath for 6–8 minutes or until cooked medium.
- At the same time, warm the cream mixture in a small saucepan, stirring over low heat for a slow, even melt.
- When the pasta is done al dente, drain and toss. Then gloss with a little olive oil and divide among four plates.
- Top the pasta with the tomato mixture.
- Gently lift the salmon out of the poaching pan and drain it. Place it atop the vegetables and pasta and then drizzle with:

  2–3 tsp fresh-squeezed lemon juice
- Pour the anchovy cream sauce over all and garnish with:

  Chopped fresh parsley

  Freshly grated Parmesan

  Fresh-ground black pepper

PESCE / FISH

HALIBUT ALLA PIZZAIOLA   (Serves 6)
Halibut Pizza Style

This is a gorgeous variation of a traditional Neapolitan red sauce that is quick to assemble and stunning enough to serve to company.

- Preheat oven to broil.
- Layer in a grill pan (from oil on bottom to onion on top):
   2 tbsp fruity olive oil
   28-oz container crushed tomatoes
   2–4 cloves garlic, slivered
   1½ lb halibut fillet, cut into 6 pieces
   12 scissored fresh basil leaves
   ½ c pitted oil-cured black olives
   1 tbsp capers
   1 medium onion, sliced thinly into rings and arranged
      over fish
- Sprinkle with:
   Sea salt, oregano and chili flakes to taste
- Drizzle with olive oil.
- Broil 10 minutes to begin charring onion. Reduce heat to 450 degrees, and bake (forno) 12–15 minutes longer.
- Serve with lemon wedges and either shards of crusty bread or a slice of hot Polenta (see recipe on p. 268).

PESCE AL CARTOCCIO   (Serves 1)
Fish Baked in Parchment

This is an amazing, complete meal in a package that can be prepared a day in advance for a no-fuss supper or easy entertaining. This recipe is for one serving; replicate it for as many people as needed. (I use this method for hassle-free cooking at even a commercial restaurant level.)

This is a master recipe. Once you grasp the concept, invent your own variations with carbohydrates (*precooked* beans, rice or potato slices), different varieties of fish, orange or lemon slices and seasonal herbs and vegetables.

- Place a 12- by 16-inch rectangle of foil (shiny side–up) on a table.
- Cover with a same-sized piece of cook's parchment paper and drizzle with a bit of olive oil.
- Lay on:
  A slab of Polenta (see recipe on p. 268)
  1 fresh bay leaf
  3–5 oz fillet of hake, haddock, pollock or similar flaky white fish
  1 slice lime
  3 oz zucchini (½ medium zucchini), sliced in ¼-inch-thick diagonals
  2 oz (¼ c) leeks, split lengthwise and chopped 1 inch long
- Drizzle with:
  1 tsp amber rum
  2 tsp olive oil
- Sprinkle with:
  Sea salt, chili flakes and dried mint
- Draw up the lengthwise sides of the foil and roll or fold edges together to form a spine. Then fold ends in a few times to seal (like rolling up a toothpaste tube).
- Preheat oven to 475–500 degrees.

- Place package on a baking sheet and bake (forno) 25–30 minutes.
- Transfer the whole package to a plate with tongs; for maximum raves, let each person open the package at the table.

TONNO CHIARO   (Serves 4)
Light Tuna Salad

Freed from the usual mayo mush, Sophia's version of this lunch staple always gets raves. Pass on the parsley, substitute tarragon for dill, add in a few capers or chopped pitted olives—this recipe is as flexible as the serving variations it suggests: Mound it on a slab of beefsteak tomato layered on a slice of Bavarian-style black rye. Serve it on a scoop of eggplant caponata for a thoroughly Sicilian taste treat. Stuff it in a Tini roll (see recipe on p. 270) spread with black olive paste, add a slice of Fontina and zap it under the broiler. Or split a Tini, drizzle the inside with olive oil and pack a summery sandwich of curly lettuce, sliced cucumber, slivered red onion and a hint of sweet and sour red pepper relish.

- Toss together in a mixing bowl:
  12-oz can solid white tuna drained well, then crumbled
  1 scallion, minced
  2 tbsp parsley leaves, chopped
  ¼ tsp dill
  ¼ tsp black pepper
  1 tbsp lemon or lime juice
  1 tbsp olive oil
  Pinch sea salt

COZZE E RISOTTO   (Serves 4)
Mussels and Risotto

Hardscrabble homesteading on the Maine coast left me with a deep
affection for two plentiful local sources of protein: mackerel and mussels. I cooked mackerel simply split and grilled over coals outdoors
with springs of oregano or thyme and drizzled with lemon. Mussels,
gathered easily from barnacled rocks at low tide, are prepared almost
as simply. My oven risotto circumvents the time-consuming traditional method. Some would argue all that stirring and gradual addition of liquid *make* it risotto, as opposed to just any old rice, but my
method provides a no-fuss alternative that also provides for the base
for another dish: cassoeula (see recipe on p. 311), a one-pot paella-like
dish that only *tastes* like you sweated over it for a long time. This oven
risotto lacks the traditional saffron, wine and cheese, but serves as a
bed for the mussels, which include all of that.

The mussels are also very nice served with a crusty baguette-style
bread, if you prefer that to risotto. Either way, accompany this with a
simple salad of fresh or grilled tomatoes and scallions and a glass of
white wine.

- Preheat oven to 400 degrees.
- In an enameled cast-iron 4-quart casserole over medium heat, stir
  together until translucent (about 2 minutes):
  1 tbsp butter
  8 oz (1⅓ c) Arborio rice
- Meanwhile, bring to a boil in a saucepan:
  3¾ c water
  ½ tsp sea salt
- Pour hot water over rice. Cover and bake (forno) 25 minutes.
- Let stand to steam, out of the oven but still covered, for 10 more
  minutes before serving. (Leave oven on to finish mussels.)
- Meanwhile, if you didn't buy cleaned mussels, scrub them to remove the beard or grassy attachment to the shell of:
  2 lb mussels

- In a large ovenproof skillet over medium heat, sauté (saltere) until onion is translucent:

  2 tbsp olive oil

  1 onion, diced

  2 cloves garlic, sliced thin

  4 bay leaves

  1 tsp fennel seed

- Add and cook until reduced (ridurre) to half:

  ½ c Italian white wine

- Add and bring to a simmer over high heat:

  8-oz (1 c) bottle clam juice

  ½ c water

  2 pinches powdered saffron

- Add mussels and *carefully* transfer to oven. Bake (forno) until mussels pop open (8–10 minutes). Discard any mussels whose shells did not open.

- Serve over plain risotto garnished with:

  Chopped parsley

  Shaved Parmesan or other hard Italian cheese

UOVE / EGGS

FRITTATA   (Serves 1)

Oven-Baked Omelet

Follow this complete meal with just a bit of fruit: a small sectioned orange or a few thin slices of melon. This is equally good as a full breakfast or dinner.

You can prepare the filling mixture in advance and store it in a plastic food-storage bag in the refrigerator for up to four days, as we do at Sophia's, making it easy to entertain or make a family brunch.

- Pierce a few times with a knife and microwave for about 4 minutes, until knife tender:
  - **1 medium (8 oz) Yukon Gold potato**
- Let stand to cool for about 5 minutes.
- Meanwhile, preheat an ovenproof 6-inch nonstick skillet in an oven set to 375–400 degrees.
- Lightly beat together and set aside:
  - **2–3 eggs**
  - **1–2 tbsp water**
- To prepare filling, combine in a bowl:
  - **2 oz (½ c) seasonal vegetable, like 6–8 5-inch-long slim asparagus spears or zucchini sliced into ¼-inch-thick diagonals**
  - **1 oz (2 tbsp) leeks or scallions, chopped into 1-inch sections**
  - **1 oz (2 tbsp) Italian cheese of choice, such as Fontina, Bel Paese, mozzarella or provolone, diced**
  - **1 oz (2 tbsp) chopped precooked meat, like capocollo ham, bacon, sausage or smoked salami (optional)**
  - **Half of the potato, cut into 1-inch cubes (reserve the other half for your next frittata)**
  - **Pinch rosemary, thyme or herb of choice**

- Pull skillet out of oven (use silicone holder). Drizzle and swirl olive oil in pan.
- Pour eggs into pan and add filling mixture.
- Bake (forno) 12–14 minutes until just set. Slide onto plate.
- Sprinkle with:
  Sea salt and pepper to taste

UOVA AL PIATTO   (Serves 4)
Baked Eggs with Beans and Salsa

Literally "plated eggs," this dish was traditionally cooked in an earthenware dish with a fresh sauce made on the spot. I've updated and simplified things a bit to give you a complete meal you can prepare and cook in under 15 minutes. The English call eggs made this way shirred, and this combination obviously takes its inspiration from Mexican *huevos rancheros*. Once you've mastered this approach, this recipe is as flexible as your imagination.

As it is here, this meal is a nutritional powerhouse. With only 370 calories, it has 24 grams of protein. But it is 30 grams shy of Diet Code recommendation for carbs, so serve it with Meini (see recipe on p. 268) or other cornbread. Or go for dessert. You could keep the Mexican theme going with Torte alla Cioccolata (see recipe on p. 316) topped with a small scoop of cinnamon gelato.

- Preheat oven and large ovenproof skillet to 400 degrees.
- Layer in the preheated skillet, in the order listed:
  20–24 oz (2½–3 c) red or green tomato salsa or other tomato sauce (or 1½ 16-oz jars)
  19-oz can red, black or white beans, drained
  8 eggs, cracked
  2 oz (½ c) shredded mozzarella
  ½ tsp oregano
- Bake (forno) 11–14 minutes or until eggs are done to your liking.
- Sprinkle with:
  Grated Parmesan

POLLO / CHICKEN

POLLO ALLA CACCIATORE   (Serves 6)
Chicken Cacciatore

This "hunter's style" dish, slow-cooked or "choked" (soffocato) to tenderness, is a one-pot meal well accompanied by hot couscous or fresh Polenta (see recipe on p. 268). This preparation is an age-old way to prepare game such as rabbit or pigeon (thus the name "hunter's style"), but modern tastes may prefer it adapted for sausage, lamb, short ribs of beef or the familiar chicken.

- Preheat oven and grill pan to 550 degrees.
- Toss together:
  3 bell peppers, cored and cut into large chunks (eighths)
  1 tbsp grapeseed oil
  1 tsp sea salt
- Roast (arrosto) 9–10 minutes until blistered and spotted with black; set aside and turn off oven.
- In stockpot, lightly brown over medium-high heat:
  2 lb mixed chicken parts
  2 fresh or 6 dried bay leaves
  2–3 cloves garlic, chopped
- Add and sauté (saltere) until golden:
  2 medium onions, cut into 1-inch chunks
- Add:
  ½ c white wine
- Reduce heat to medium-low. Cover and stew for 30 minutes, adding up to ½ c water as necessary to retain liquid.
- Add:
  28-oz container crushed tomatoes
  2–3 tbsp tomato paste
  1 tbsp turbinado sugar

½ **tsp sea salt**

8–12 sage leaves, torn

4 carrots, peeled and cut into 2- to 3-inch lengths

- Stew over medium-low heat for 1 hour with cover slightly ajar. (Optional: Add 2 stalks of celery cut into 2- to 3-inch lengths after 40 minutes.)
- Remove from heat and add peppers.
- Let stand 15–20 minutes before serving.
- Garnish with:

Grated Parmesan or other hard Italian cheese

POLLO AI LIMONI (Serves 6)

Lemon Chicken

North African influenced, this dish is great made ahead and served cold for picnics or as an impromptu meal with a salad and bread or couscous. It has appetizing black and yellow striping from the saffron and the grill pan.

- A day ahead, rinse and pat dry, and place in a 1-gallon plastic food-storage bag:

2 lb mixed chicken pieces

- Mix marinade:

Zest and juice of ½ lemon

3 cloves garlic, crushed

2 tsp black olive paste or crushed capers

2 tsp olive oil

2 pinches saffron powder

½ tsp chili flakes

½ tsp dried mint or thyme

½ tsp turmeric

- Add to bag with chicken, toss to coat, and let marinate in refrigerator overnight.

• Preheat oven and grill pan to 450 degrees.
• Sear (salto) chicken skin side–down for 12 minutes.
• Reduce heat to 400 degrees.
• Turn chicken pieces with tongs. Sprinkle with sea salt and bake (forno) 15 minutes longer or until the internal temperature of the chicken reaches 170 degrees.

SALSICCE E FAGIOLI   (Serves 4)
Chicken Sausage and Beans

This oven-baked dish provides authentic Italian flavor in 30 minutes. I make it often with chicken sausage, but you can substitute orange-scented locanico (Greek sausage) or your favorite sweet or hot Italian sausage. Serve with Braised Broccolini or Broccoli Raab (see recipe on p. 288) topped with grated Parmesan or other hard Italian cheese.

• Preheat oven and grill pan to broil.
• Sear (salto) 12 oz (4 links) organic chicken sausage for 3–4 minutes.
• Reduce oven to 400 degrees.
• Sauté (saltere) in ovenproof enameled cast-iron casserole on stove top:
    2 tbsp olive oil
    3 cloves garlic, chopped
    1 onion, diced
    **2 carrots, peeled and sliced into ½-inch-thick diagonals
        2 inches long**
    6–8 sage leaves
    2 bay leaves
    ½ tsp fennel seeds
• Add:
    19-oz can butter beans or cannellini beans, undrained
    2 c chicken broth (or 2 c water and 1 cube or 1 tsp bouillon)
    Broiled sausage
• Bake (forno) 20 minutes.

CARNE / MEAT

SPADE DI MANZO (Serves 4)

Skewered Short Ribs

This is a Tuscan-style grill that maximizes the flavor of a very inexpensive cut of beef. It is easily accompanied by rice and a sauté of mushrooms and summer squash, or a sweet potato and buttered spinach. Or slice it up "fajita style" and pile it into a hot pita with roasted peppers. The meat really needs to sit in the marinade, so you'll want to put this together the day before you plan to cook it—or at least in the morning for that night's supper. Thinking ahead will be more than worth it when you see how fragrant and juicy the beef will be.

- 8–24 hours ahead of time, combine in a large food-storage bag:
  1 tbsp olive oil
  3 tbsp hickory BBQ sauce
  1 tsp aged balsamic vinegar
  1 tsp fresh oregano leaves
  ½ tsp cracked black pepper
  ¼ tsp ground coriander or ½ tsp coriander seeds
  Pinch ground clove
- Place in bag, seal and store in the refrigerator:
  1 lb (4 strips) boneless beef short ribs
- Half an hour before cooking, prepare outdoor grill or preheat oven and grill pan to 550 degrees.
- Thread each strip of beef onto a bamboo skewer.
- Grill (brace) 5 minutes on each side, using tongs to turn.

AGNELLO ALL 'ACETO   (Serves 4)
Lamb Stew

A unique combination of grilling and stewing produces a dish with very complex flavorings from the bacon, rum, prunes, clove and red wine vinegar (from which it gets the name *aceto*), yet it's very straightforward to prepare. It shines with equally straightforward accompaniments, like pastina—tiny acini di pepe or stellete pasta—and baby fingerling carrots braised with butter and sage.

- Preheat oven and grill pan to broil.
- Whisk together and set aside:
    1 c water
    2 tsp flour (preferably spelt)
    1 tsp mushroom stock concentrate
    1 tbsp amber rum
- Combine in bowl and set aside:
    2 strips bacon, cut into 1-inch pieces
    2 medium onions, cut in 1-inch, squarish chunks
    8 prunes, pitted
    6-oz package crimini mushrooms, brushed clean and halved
    2 cloves garlic, thickly sliced
    1 tsp capers
    1 tbsp olive oil
- Toss to coat in a large food-storage bag:
    1 lb lamb sirloin strips or cubed stew meat
    ½ tsp black pepper
    ½ tsp rosemary
    ¼ tsp ground clove
- Arrange lamb in a single layer in grill pan and broil for 6 minutes without turning.
- Add bacon and onion mix and broil 4 more minutes without turning.
- Reduce oven to 375 degrees.

- Add to pan and return to oven for 5 minutes to deglaze:

  ¼ c red wine vinegar

- Stir and add stock mixture. Cover grill pan with a baking sheet and stew in the oven 20–25 minutes, or until thickened. Serve immediately.

CASSOEULA (Serves 4)

Pork Sausage Casserole

The term *casserole* evolved from the Greek word for ladle—*kyathos*. This version updates and lightens the traditional savoy cabbage and pork dish (originally featuring the skin, ribs and feet along with the sausage), from the Lombard region of Leonardo's patron Sforza, to a one-pot feast recalling a Spanish paella.

- Preheat oven to 400 degrees.
- In a 4-quart ovenproof, cast-iron casserole over medium heat, brown:

  8 oz pork sausage (plain or spicy), cut into 1-inch chunks

- Add to casserole and sauté until translucent, 2–3 minutes:

  8 oz (1⅓ c) long grain brown rice

  2 fresh or 6 dried bay leaves

  2 pinches saffron or ¼ tsp smoked paprika

- Meanwhile, bring to a boil in a saucepan over high heat:

  2 c chicken stock or 2 c water plus 1 cube bouillon

- Pour broth over rice and bring to a boil. Then add in layers in the order listed:

  4 oz (¼ lb) large, raw peeled shrimp

  10- to 12-oz package whole gold or red cherry tomatoes

  10 oz (4 c) savoy cabbage, in ¼-inch-wide slices

  2 scallions, cut into 2-inch lengths

  ½ c parsley leaves

  2 tbsp olive oil

  ½ tsp anise or caraway seeds

- Cover, transfer to oven and bake (forno) 40 minutes. Remove from oven and let stand for 10 minutes before "ladling" into bowls.

DOLCE / DESSERT

BUDINO   (Serves 4–6)
Chocolate Pudding

Budino is a nontraditional, dairy-free chocolate "mousse" that will charm even most mainstream dessert buffs. Tell them the secret ingredient to show them you care about their health. The pudding will keep in the refrigerator for up to four days.

- In a blender or food processor, puree:
    10-oz package silken tofu (do not use regular tofu)
    1 tbsp maple syrup
    1–2 tsp rum
    1–2 tbsp coffee (or 1 tsp instant coffee dissolved in 2 tbsp water)
    ½ tsp vanilla or orange flower water
    ¼ tsp almond extract (optional)
- Melt in microwave, about 1–1½ minutes:
    6 oz (1 c) bittersweet chocolate chips, like Ghirardelli
- Pulse chocolate into tofu mix until mousselike.
- Spoon into ramekins or custard cups and chill to set, about 1–2 hours.

FICHI PIGNATI   (Serves 4)
Poached Figs

One of the simplest and most ancient desserts, this dish is every bit as intriguing today as it must have been 2,500 years ago.

- In a saucepan over medium heat, dissolve:
    ½ c water
    ½ c turbinado sugar or honey

1 c zinfandel *or* other red wine

- Add:

    6 oz (1 c) organic black mission figs (or pitted prunes)

    ¼ orange or lemon (to be removed later) or 1 tbsp orange
    marmalade

- Spice with just one or two of the following options:

    1 cinnamon stick

    ¼ tsp aniseed or fennel seed

    A few whole peppercorns, allspice berries, cloves or coriander
    seeds

- Cover and poach until tender, 20–30 minutes.
- Remove and set aside fruit.
- Strain liquid remaining in the pan, then return to heat and reduce
  (ridurre) to a thick syrup over medium heat.
- Serve figs alongside:

    ¼ c ricotta, buffalo milk yogurt, Crema di Mascarpone (see
    recipe below) or rich ice cream

- Drizzle with the syrup reduced from the poaching liquid, and
  sprinkle on:

    2 tsp almonds, walnuts, pine nuts or pistachios, warmed or
    toasted

CREMA DI MASCARPONE (Serves 6)

Mascarpone Cream

A voluptuous substitute for ice cream or whipped cream developed from
a rich Italian soft cheese, this can accompany fresh berries, melon or
poached fruit, or can be piped into cannoli tubes or puff pastry shells.

- Beat with electric mixer until the consistency of soft whipped cream:

    8 oz mascarpone cheese

    2 oz (½ c) confectioner's sugar

    1 tbsp liquor

    ½ tsp flavor extract

- If accompanying with fresh strawberries, use brandy, vanilla *and* almond extracts, and then sprinkle with sliced almonds.
- To use with Fichi Pignati (see recipe on p. 312) or fresh blueberries or melon, use brandy or anisette and add 1 teaspoon of lemon zest.
- For a zabaglione flavor that mates well with cherries, use rum *and* marsala, as well as 1 teaspoon of lemon zest.

NICOLLETTA   (Serves 1)
Hasty Bread Pudding

Though this is definitely not just for kids, even four-year-olds can make this for themselves. If you preslice the bread, they can cube it with a safe table knife. For extra nutrition, use a multigrain loaf with millet pieces, pumpkinseed, sunflower, flax and sesame seed.

- Toss together gently in a microwave-safe bowl:
  1 oz (½-inch slice) multigrain bread cut into 1-inch squares
  ⅓ c soy milk or milk
  1 tbsp raisins
  1 tbsp honey
  ⅛ tsp cinnamon
- Microwave for 1 minute and serve immediately.

TORTA DI SEMI   (Serves 16)
Seedcake

This wayfarer's bread unites seven seeds representing Fundamental Food sources from all continents in a perfect Fibonacci progression by weight. It's inspired by the famed *panforte* of Siena, Tuscany, the "strong bread" of spiced honey, nut and citrus peel carried by the Crusaders. This recipe forms the Fibonacci sequence:

$$\frac{1 + 1 + 2 + 3 + 5 + 8 + 13 + 21}{2}$$

- Preheat oven to 350 degrees.
- Oil and lightly flour an 8-inch or 9-inch, removable-bottom, round cake pan.
- Measure, toss together and set aside:

  2 tbsp (½ oz) amaranth (or quinoa) flour

  2 tbsp (½ oz) poppy seeds

  3 tbsp (1 oz) hemp seeds

  ¼ c (1½ oz) golden flaxseeds

  ½ c (2½ oz) pumpkin seeds

  ¾ c (4 oz) sesame seeds

  1¼ c (6½ oz) sunflower seeds

  1 tsp coriander

  ½ tsp cinnamon

  ¼ tsp white pepper

- In a saucepan over medium heat, simmer (sobollire) for 5–8 minutes to thicken:

  15 tbsp (10½ oz by weight, or 220 ml—just short of 1 c) honey

  1 tsp orange flower water

  1 tsp vanilla

- Fold honey mixture into seed mix and scrape into pan.
- Wet hands, then press dough flat.
- Bake (forno) 35 minutes or until golden.
- Cool for six hours, pry out of pan and cut into 16 wedges.

TORRONE DI SARDEGNA   (Makes 16 2½-inch squares)

Almond Nougat

This very nutritious, chewy nut confection from Sardinia is flourless and wheat-free, best made in fall and winter under low humidity.

- Preheat oven to 350 degrees.
- Toss together:

  12 oz (3¾ c) sliced almonds

   1 tbsp cornstarch

   Pinch baking soda

- Heat in a saucepan over medium heat until just simmering:

   ¼ c turbinado sugar

   2 tbsp orange marmalade

   1 tbsp honey

   1 tsp rosewater (or orange flower water)

- Fold hot syrup into nuts.
- Spread in well-buttered or oiled 10- by 10-inch cake pan.
- Bake (forno) 15–18 minutes or until amber but not brown.
- Cool 15–20 minutes and score into squares immediately (or cool thoroughly and snap into irregular pieces).

TORTE ALLA CIOCCOLATA   (Serves 6)

Chocolate Cakes

This lush, flourless rum chocolate indulgence is breathtakingly simple and elegant. Serve hot and molten with cold Italian cherry (amarena) preserves, a dusting of powdered sugar, shaved almonds and a mint leaf for the ultimate rush.

Cakes will keep 3–5 days at room temperature; reheat in microwave for about 30 seconds to restore molten centers.

- Preheat oven to 350 degrees.
- Fit a 6-cup "Texas-sized" muffin mold with paper liners, then spray with food-release cooking spray.
- Microwave 1½ minutes and set aside:

   8 oz (1⅓ c) dark Italian chocolate chips (like Ghirardelli)

   ⅓ c light olive oil

- Beat until creamy:

   3 eggs

   ½ c turbinado sugar

   2 tbsp amber rum

1 tsp instant coffee
1 tsp vanilla extract
1 oz (⅓ c) unsweetened cocoa
½ tsp baking powder
⅛ tsp baking soda
½ tsp cinnamon

- Beat in melted chocolate until smooth and glossy.
- Portion evenly into muffin cups.
- Bake (forno) 24–25 minutes until fully puffed and cracking open (will fall slightly when cooling because of soft centers).

BRUTTI   (Makes 10 meringues)

"Ugly" Meringues

These frumpy, flourless, Milanese-style treats are a pure Italian confection. Crisp, pale brown exteriors hide a chewy cocoa brownie-like interior studded with nuts. They are best aged for a day or two after baking.

Look for orange flower water in your supermarket or Italian or Middle Eastern market. This is an ancient flavoring more widely used before vanilla was available (although they don't taste anything alike).

- Preheat oven to 350 degrees.
- Pulse in a food processor until pea sized and set aside:
    4 oz (1¼ c) pistachios or walnuts
    1½ oz (⅓ c) confectioners' sugar
    1 oz (⅓ c) unsweetened cocoa
    ⅛ tsp baking soda
- Fork together until blended and set aside:
    4 oz (½ c) cane sugar
    1 tbsp cornstarch
    ½ tsp orange flower water
- Whip until soft and foamy:
    3 egg whites

- Slowly add in sugar mix and beat until glossy and stiff, about 5 minutes.
- Fold in nut mix by hand to barely blend together (do not overmix and make smooth).
- Dollop with a tablespoon onto sprayed cook's parchment on baking sheet.
- Bake (forno) 25–30 minutes.

TORTA CONTADINA (Serves 16)
Rum Raisin Country Cake

This is a moist, rich, wheat-free whole grain spice cake good with coffee for breakfast or as an afternoon treat.

- Preheat oven to 350 degrees.
- Spray or oil a 10- by 10-inch cake pan.
- Beat together:
    4 eggs
    1 c light olive oil or sunflower oil
    1 c honey
    2 tbsp rum
    1 tsp vanilla extract
    12 oz (2 c) raisins (mixed golden and black is nice), dried currants or diced dried apricots
- Whisk together, then fold into egg mix:
    8 oz whole rye flour
    3 oz whole spelt flour
    1 tsp cocoa
    1 tsp instant coffee
    1 tsp cinnamon
    1 tsp coriander
    1 tsp ground black pepper
    1 tbsp plus 1 tsp baking powder
- Pour into pan and spread batter evenly.

- Bake (forno) 40–50 minutes.
- Cool and then cut into sixteen 2½-inch squares.
- For a little decadence, drizzle with a tablespoon of amber rum or marsala and accompany with a ¼-cup scoop of chilled ricotta sprinkled with nutmeg, demerara sugar crystals and soft sautéed sliced peaches.

SBRICIOLONA (Makes 16 cookies)

Crumb Cookies

I've turned a traditional Tuscan spiced almond cornmeal-crumb cookie into a granola-like square that's 25 percent old bread!

- Preheat oven to 325 degrees.
- Spray a 10- by 10-inch cake pan with food-release cooking spray.
- Beat in a small dish with fork and reserve:
  1 egg
  ⅓ c sunflower oil
  ½ tsp almond extract
  ½ tsp vanilla extract
- Pulse to pea size in a food processor:
  4 oz (1¼ c) fine unflavored breadcrumbs (whole grain preferred)
  4 oz (1¼ c) sliced almonds
  4 oz (1¼ c) walnuts
  4 oz (1¼ c) rolled oats or 2 oz (⅔ c) rolled oats and 2 oz (⅓ c) cornmeal
  ½ c demerara sugar
  ½ tsp cinnamon
  ½ tsp coriander
  ¼ tsp baking soda
- Stir egg mixture into crumbs with a fork and blend well.
- Loosely shake mix into pan, and lightly pat flat.

- Bake (forno) 35 minutes.
- Cut into 16 squares within 5 minutes after baking *or* let cool completely and break into irregular pieces.

FRUTTO E FORMAGGIO
Fruit and Cheese

This might be the sort of thing a baker isn't supposed to confess, but this most ancient Italian dessert is still, to be honest, my favorite. Not in the American form of dismal commercially processed cheeses and fruit carted about in trucks for who knows how long before landing in the store, to be sure! But the simple pairing of ripe, local fruit and artisanal cheese is most often the way I *really* want to finish a meal. So, this "recipe" is just some suggested pairings inspired by traditional Italian choices. Serve each person 1 ounce of cheese and 6 ounces of fresh fruit—¾ cup berries, or 1 large or 2 small pieces of whole fruit. For dried fruit, serve 1½ ounces, or ¼ cup.

- Caciotta del Lazio (soft sheep's milk) and dried figs
- Piave Vecchio (a nutty hard cheese) and apples
- Vento d'estate (hard grainy cheese cured in—and tasting of—hay) and pear
- Pecorino Pepato (peppercorn-studded sheep's milk) and black grapes
- Gorgonzola dolcelatte (sweet milk blue-veined cheese) and cantaloupe
- Stracchino (soft sweet "young" paper-wrapped cow's milk) and peach or Mostarda di Cremona, a traditional spiced fruit relish
- Ricotta and raspberries, blackberries or sliced strawberries. (You can fancy this up by dripping ½ teaspoon artisanal balsamic vinegar on the berries and sprinkling 1–2 teaspoons coarse demerara sugar crystals on ¼ cup fresh ricotta.)

FIVE-COURSE FEAST   (Serves 6)

The Diet Code is meant to be everyday food, but that doesn't mean you can't whip up a festive meal—worthy of company and the good china—when you want to. Best of all, you can still make it quick in the kitchen. I've laid out a series of interlocking recipes here to get the whole spread on the table *in one hour*.

Though it could work for any occasion, especially during cool weather, as you might guess, this menu was originally designed to be Thanksgiving dinner. (Thanksgiving—in an hour!) This is my Italian twist on this most American of holidays. (Or is it an American twist on an Italian menu?)

Serve the soup first, then combine the next three "courses" American style by composing each plate before bringing it to the table. The turkey with the deep green kale and the bright red cranberry sauce is very festive looking and is rightly accompanied by a pinot nero wine. Follow up the meal with fresh-piped cannoli and coffee.

MENU

Purea di Carciofi (Cream of Artichoke Soup)
Tacchino Arrosto (Roast Turkey Thighs)
Salsa D'Agresto Bollito (Cranberry Sauce)
Cavolo Nero Brasato (Braised Black Kale)
Cannoli di Zucca (Pumpkin Cannoli)

Stage 1: Cannoli di Zucca (10 minutes)

• *Preheat grill pan for turkey in oven at 450 degrees.*
• Combine in mixer and beat until thick, like stiff whipped cream:
    8 oz (1 c) ricotta
    8 oz (1 c) mascarpone
    8 oz (1 c) pumpkin or winter squash puree (canned organic works well)

    4 oz (1 c) confectioners' sugar

    1 tbsp rum or brandy

    ¼ tsp vanilla

    1 tsp lemon zest

    ½ tsp each cinnamon, nutmeg and ginger

- Scrape filling into pastry bag fitted with a star tip and set aside in refrigerator.
- Just before serving, pipe into prepared cannoli shells and dust with confectioners' sugar mixed with cinnamon.

Stage 2: Tacchino Arrosto (40 minutes)

- Rinse and place in preheated grill pan skin side–down:

    6 turkey thighs

- Add:

    2–3 tbsp water to keep from smoking

- Roast (arrosto) for 15 minutes; baste with drippings, turn over, and roast 10 more minutes.
- Baste with drippings, then brush on glaze made of:

    ¼ c hickory BBQ sauce

    ¼ c Tuscan bilberry (or wild blueberry) preserves

- Roast (arrosto) 5–7 more minutes to color and bubble glaze.
- Remove from oven, cover with a foil tent, and let stand 10–12 minutes before serving.

Stage 3: Salsa D'Agresto Bollito (15 minutes, while turkey is roasting)

This spice combination will bring you back to the Renaissance.

- Combine in a saucepan and bring to a simmer:

    6 oz raw cranberries (half of a standard 12-oz package)

    2 oz (⅓ c) pitted prunes, halved

½ c water
½ c orange marmalade
2-inch sprig rosemary
Cracked black pepper to taste

• Simmer (sobollire) 10 minutes, remove from heat, and allow to thicken before serving.

Stage 4: Purea di Carciofi (15 minutes, while turkey is roasting)

• In a blender or food processor, puree and set aside:
    4 oz artichoke hearts (half of a 14-oz can, drained)
    3 mint leaves
    1 c cream
• In a saucepan, bring to a simmer:
    1 c chicken stock (*or* 1 c water plus ½ cube or 1 tsp chicken boullion)
    1 tbsp rum
• Poach for 30–40 seconds on each side:
    6 fresh jumbo shrimp (peeled and deveined)
• Remove shrimp from broth and place one in each serving bowl.
• Stream broth into cream, then strain back into saucepan and reheat until scalding (do not boil, or it will curdle).
• Ladle ¼ cup over each shrimp, and garnish each bowl with:
    1 mint leaf
    A few drops of peppery olive oil
    Chili flakes to taste

Stage 5: Cavolo Nero Brasato (10 minutes, while turkey is standing under foil)

• Wash, destem and slice ⅜ inch wide:
    24 oz (6 c) black or lacinato kale

- Toss in bowl or plastic food-storage bag with:
    ¼ c olive oil
    2–4 tbsp water
    6 cloves garlic, sliced
- Preheat large skillet over medium heat.
- Braise greens 4–5 minutes, or until just tender.
- Add sea salt and pepper to taste and serve immediately.

APPENDIX A

Golden Macronutrient Profiles

The following chart lists the macronutrient profiles of some of the most common Diet Code foods. It gives you the hard numbers first (how many calories and how many grams of carbs, protein and fat) and then the ratios (percentage of calories from carbs, protein and fat). Remember: You should aim to get 52% of your calories from carbs, 20% from protein and 28% from fat. There are 4 calories per gram of carbohydrate, 4 calories per gram of protein and 9 calories per gram of fat. There isn't room in this book for a comprehensive listing of every nutritional component of every food you might ever eat while on The Diet Code, of course, but this should be sufficient to help you work out the Golden Ratio in your own meals or recipes or see how changes you make to my menus or recipes affect the total counts and the balances between them.

You won't need to do this every day if you are using the menu plans in chapter 9. But when you want to create your own meals and menus, convert a family favorite to meet the Golden Ratio, check out your usual breakfast or your regular lunch take-out order or just get some hands-on experience in the nitty-gritty of how The Diet Code comes together, this is the place to turn for reference. This chart can also help you troubleshoot your technique if you've hit a snag and are not losing weight or are doing so at too slow a pace for your liking. Those are signs that you are off balance somewhere, despite all your efforts, and your body requires more precisely measured foods to respond. You can pin down what estimation or substitution you made that got you off course so you can get right back on.

Perhaps most valuably, the three columns of percentages—calories from carb, protein and fat—give you a quick idea of the primary energy source of a particular food. Getting familiar with what you are eating—appreciating each food and what it can do—is the best way to help you improvise your own Diet Code meals intuitively. Here, what you observe will reinforce the arrangement of the five food groups, which are grouped according to dominant macronutrient. You'll also be able to see, even within a category, what the strongest sources of the dominant macronutrient are. Calorie for calorie, you get a lot more protein from tuna or halibut, for example, than you do from steak or lamb. In addition, you'll notice that certain dairy products (like buttermilk, ricotta and especially Parmesan) and beans and seeds (lentils, tempeh and hemp) rival red meats in their caloric profiles for protein. Finally, with this chart you'll be able to find components in foods that might surprise you, like the protein percentage (by calories) in greens.

To give you perspective on the information in the long chart below, here again is the summary of ideal Golden Ratio proportions at various calorie levels.

DIET CODE MACRONUTRIENT PROFILES			
Calories	Carbohydrates (in grams)	Protein (in grams)	Fat (in grams)
100	13	5	3
200	25	10	6
300	38	15	9
400	51	19	12
500	64	24	15
600	76	29	18
700	89	34	21

MACRONUTRIENT PROFILE AND CALORIE COUNTS OF COMMON FOODS

(Based on data in *Nutrition Almanac,* fifth edition, by Lavon Dunne, and on food labels.)

FATTY PROTEINS (FP)									
Food	ounces	measure	cal	carb (g)	pro (g)	fat (g)	carb (%)	pro (%)	fat (%)
Butter	½	½ tbsp	99	–	–	11	–	–	100
Olive oil	½	1 tbsp	126	–	–	14	–	–	100
Chocolate, dark	¾		99	–	–	11	–	–	100
Bacon	½	1 strip	67	–	1	7	–	6	94
Mascarpone	1	2 tbsp	125	–	2	13	–	6	94
Olive	2	8–10	49	1	5	–	–	8	92
Sour cream	1	2 tbsp	62	1	1	6	6	6	88
Cream	1	2 tbsp	102	1	2	10	4	8	88
Avocado	2	¼ fruit	79	3	1	7	15	5	80
Half-and-half	2½	¼ c	79	2	2	7	10	10	80
Mozzarella, fresh	2		140	–	8	12	–	23	77
Nut/seed	1	¼ c	170	4	7	14	9	16	75
Provolone/ Fontina	1		109	–	7	9	–	26	74
Peanut butter	1	2 tbsp	192	5	8	16	10	16	74
Flaxseed	½	2 tbsp	95	5	3	7	21	13	66
Parmesan, grated		1 tbsp	23	–	2	< 2	–	35	65
Ricotta	2	¼ c	110	3	7	8	10	25	65
Hemp seed meal	1	3 tbsp	135	9	14	< 5	27	41	32

LEAN PROTEINS (LP)

Food	ounces	measure	cal	carb (g)	pro (g)	fat (g)	carb (%)	pro (%)	fat (%)
Haddock	3		73	–	16	1	–	88	12
Halibut	3		90	–	18	2	–	80	20
Scallop	3		73	2	14	1	11	77	12
Tuna	3		107	–	20	3	–	75	25
Shrimp	3		104	–	17	4	–	65	35
Turkey/ chicken	3		139	–	19	7	–	55	45
Cottage cheese	3		88	2	11	4	9	50	41
Chicken sausage	3	1 link	105	3	12	5	11	46	43
Tempeh	4	½ package	192	12	18	8	25	38	37
Smoked salmon	2		129	–	12	9	–	37	63
Lamb	3		168	–	15	12	–	36	64
Steak	3		224	–	20	16	–	36	64
Egg	3	2 large	137	2	12	9	6	35	59
Sardine	3		151	–	13	11	–	34	66

STARCHY PROTEINS (SP)

Food	ounces	measure	cal	carb (g)	pro (g)	fat (g)	carb (%)	pro (%)	fat (%)
Sweet potato	8	1 c	216	51	3	–	94	6	–
Potato, white	8	1 c	184	41	5	–	89	11	–

Food	ounces	measure	cal	carb (g)	pro (g)	fat (g)	carb (%)	pro (%)	fat (%)
Corn, fresh	8	1 c	212	46	7	–	87	13	–
Kidney bean	8	1 c	225	40	14	1	71	25	4
Lentil	8	1 c	225	39	15	1	69	27	4
Chickpea	8	1 c	267	45	15	3	67	22	11
Bean spread	4	½ c	241	32	8	9	53	13	34
Buttermilk/ Kvass	8	1 c	98	12	8	2	49	33	18
Yogurt/Kefir	8	1 c	133	13	9	5	39	27	34
Beer, premium	12		146	13	< 1	–	36	–	–
Soy milk	8	1 c	110	9	7	5	33	25	42
Wine, red	5		106	2	–	–	8	–	–

GRAINS (G)

Most whole grain products—whether bread, crackers, pasta, rice or unsweetened cereals (100% cracked or rolled grains)—all show a generally uniform nutritional profile.

Food	ounces	measure	cal	carb (g)	pro (g)	fat (g)	carb (%)	pro (%)	fat (%)
Whole grains	2 (dry)	⅓ c	190– 210	35– 40	5– 8	2– 4	75 (avg)	14 (avg)	11 (avg)
Sprouted grain tortilla	2	two 6-inch rounds	160	29	6	2	73	15	12
Westphalian/ Bavarian whole meal sourdough bread	2	one ⅜-inch-thick, 4-inch-square slice	138	25	5	2	73	15	12

VEGETABLES AND FRUITS (VF)
VEGETABLES

Food	ounces	measure	cal	carb (g)	pro (g)	fat (g)	carb (%)	pro (%)	fat (%)
Cauliflower Green bean Pepper Tomato sauce	5	¾–1 c	35	8	< 2	–	**92**	8	–
Parsnip Winter squash	5	¾–1 c	84	18	3	–	**86**	14	–
Dandelion greens Onion	5	¾–1 c	50	10	< 3	–	**80**	20	–
Brussels sprout Pumpkin	5	¾–1 c	60	12	3	–	**80**	20	–
Beet Carrot Chard Kale Leek Parsley	5	¾–1 c	68	13	4	–	**76**	24	–
Arugula Asparagus Broccoli Cabbage Collard greens Mushroom Mustard greens Sauerkraut	5	¾–1 c	40	7	3	–	**70**	30	–

FRUITS

Food	ounces	measure	cal	carb (g)	pro (g)	fat (g)	carb (%)	pro (%)	fat (%)
Honey Molasses	¼	1 tbsp	68	17	–	–	**100**	–	–
Raw sugar		1 tbsp	45	11	–	–	**100**	–	–

Food	ounces	measure	cal	carb (g)	pro (g)	fat (g)	carb (%)	pro (%)	fat (%)
Fig Prune Raisin	1½	½ c	116	28	1	–	97	3	–
Apple Pear	5	¾–1 c	84	21	< 1	–	97	3	–
Banana Grape	5	¾–1 c	92	22	1	–	96	4	–
Blueberry	5	¾–1 c	88	21	1	< 1	95	5	–
Orange Peach	5	¾–1 c	64	15	1	–	94	6	–
Blackberry Plum Raspberry	5	¾–1 c	72	17	1	–	94	6	–
Cantaloupe Strawberry	5	¾–1 c	52	12	< 2	–	92	8	–

APPENDIX B

Golden Ratio Math and Myth

A footprint left in damp earth was likely the first mark left by early man, closely followed by the impression of a hand—much like the plaster of Paris plaques schoolchildren stamp with their little clusters of digits. This five-fingered imprint became the mark of man, appearing the same as our five-pointed body outline of head with spread-eagle arms and legs. Our ancestors associated self-semblance with natural forms that exhibited fiveness, especially the wild rose (in its petal arrangement) and the apple. Cut an apple sideways through its core. The seeds form a five-pointed star bound by a circle, which we call a pentacle. Sameness of form provided early man with a sense of order and a way to derive meaning from nature and the cosmos.

By 1490, while he was still in the Milan of Sforza, Leonardo completed a pen and ink drawing that graphically illustrated this handprint, or autograph, of man. His *Vitruvian Man* was dedicated to the Roman architect and military engineer Marcus Vitruvius Pollio, who advocated that well-proportioned body measure should be, in turn, applied to buildings and civic projects for optimal function and beauty.

Pollio's stance was supported by the ancient universal use of the body as the initial source of measure, in fingers, hands, feet and arm's reach. Proportions of the body—the interrelationship between body parts—first sized tools, weapons and shelter, but expanded seamlessly beyond "home ergonomics" to public buildings and temples, then to the division of land as communal complexity grew.

Ancient body measures have been much maligned for their inherent irregularity (each body is so different), especially since the standardization of the metric system in the eighteenth century based on modern measure of the earth's surface, supposedly without regard to the size of man.

But the flaws in ancient systems have more to do with the fact that, through the ages, they have been mixed up, modified and recombined. In the United States, our feet, yards and miles are British adaptations of early Roman measures. The word *mile,* which comes from the Latin term *mille passus,* meant a thousand paces. In Roman times, a mile was 5,000 feet, but our present British imperial unit has grown to 5,280 feet.

The Egyptians, however, produced a geometric correlation between the human hand and celestial bodies to devise their measure of length, the cubit, and their measure of angle or slope, the *sekhed.* So precise was their "hand jive" reckoning that it has been demonstrated to predict the orbital periods of the earth, moon, Venus and Mars.

THE GREAT PYRAMID

The uncanny accuracy of ancient body measurements is nowhere better represented than at 30 degrees N latitude (exactly halfway between the equator and the north pole) and 30 degrees E Rose Line longitude (now 31 degrees E Greenwich). Built during the fourth Egyptian dynasty in the reign of Khufu (about 2,550 BCE), the colossal five-sided Great Pyramid is the most massive edifice ever constructed (short of the Great Wall of China). Dating of mortar samples places construction over a period of about 85 years, carried out by rotating conscripted workforces of 20,000 "carb junkies" fueled by bread and beer. Quarried stones weighing up to 70 tons each were lifted and fitted with the accuracy of a luxury car door to construct a pyramid almost 500 feet high.

The miraculous engineering was attributed to a demiurge named Thoth (pronounced tōt), a grand archon, or architect of math, sciences and music. So complete was his influence that the subsequent Latin word *totus* became our word *total*! Reminders of the name of this mover of stones linger also in several African dialects (meaning to pile up, bear or carry) from which we borrow our word *tote*. The Greeks renamed Thoth Hermes (from the Greek *herma*, meaning pile of stones).

The Great Pyramid is claimed to be a matrix of mathematical secrets, containing precise encoded measures of the size, mass, density, elemental makeup and destiny of both earth and man. Bread was so significant to the pyramid builders and indeed to all Egyptians that it is the only hieroglyph found in the Great Pyramid. Their mark for bread (like the letter D) was carved into the Granite Leaf Seal (sliding stone door) sealing the king's chambers. This half circle, resembling the cross section of a loaf of artisanal bread or a domed baker's oven,

---

PYTHAGOREAN HARMONIES AND THE IRRATIONAL NUMBER PHI

A rational number can be expressed as a simple ratio of integers, like 1:2 (one half). An irrational number can't.

Simple ratios gave rise to a basic musical scale supposedly discovered by Pythagoras of Samos (500 BCE), who picked up on the harmonious ring of blacksmiths' hammers cast in regular weights (1, 2, 3 and 4 units or pounds).

1:1 is unison, a mirror image.
2:1 is the octave (a double).
3:2 is the fifth.
4:3 is the fourth.
The fourth and fifth together re-form the octave:
$$4/3 \times 3/2 = 12/6 \text{ or } 2:1$$

(continued on next page)

Adding weights of 5 and 6 expands the harmonic possibilities:
5:4 is the major third.
6:5 is the minor third.

Expressed as fractions, they appear:

Rational Harmonies	Their Reciprocal Ratios
1:1 = 1	itself
2:1 = 2	1:2 = ½ = 0.5
3:2 = ³⁄₂ = 1.5	2:3 = ⅔ = 0.66̄
4:3 = ⁴⁄₃ = 1.33̄	3:4 = ¾ = 0.75
5:4 = ⁵⁄₄ = 1.25	4:5 = ⅘ = 0.8
6:5 = ⁶⁄₅ = 1.2	5:6 = ⁵⁄₆ = 0.83̄

These reciprocal ratios can be used to make bread formulae.

With rational numbers, even though some of the fractional values repeat (1.3̄), they do so regularly and measurably. Whether expressed in hammer or bell weights or chime or string lengths, they sound nice and harmonious and track straight.

Irrational numbers don't. Phi approximates 1.6180339887 . . . It wavers. It doesn't walk the line. And that's its paradoxical value; by turning, bending and diverging from the straight path, *phi can create formulae for curves.*

is an ancient symbol of stored potential—like a strung bow or the profile of a mother-to-be.

Built over two millennia before modern mathematicians are comfortable admitting the discovery of irrational numbers, the Golden Pyramid (it once had a gold capstone) nonetheless encodes the most compelling one: phi. Most of us will never directly utilize this value (until you start eating The Diet Code way!), and yet we encounter it hundreds of times a day.

If your cat's scratched you or if you've ever paddled a surfboard, you've had a run-in with phi. Phi determines natural curves, from claws to ocean waves. The pyramid incorporates this factor for curves into a straight-sided stone structure weighing over 5 million tons that's 30 times the mass of the Empire State Building. Both the ratio of the area of the pyramid's sides to its base and the proportion of the length of its slope to half its base exhibit phi. Perfectly? No. There are 5 million tons of rock there, after all. However, it approaches phi with an accuracy of 99.9%.

Ancient structures like pyramids show an unavoidable and declarative geometry that is again highly visible in the works of Renaissance artists. There's a geometric redundancy that somehow *bends* our attention to them. And this bending or attraction may be the result of the mysterious property of phi.

MESSENGER ANGLES OF THE PENTACLE

From Giotto (1267–1337, generally considered the progenitor of the Renaissance) and Piero della Francesca (1420–1492, whose paintings display an eerie, almost disconcerting angularity) to Leonardo and on to Tintoretto at the end of the sixteenth century, much attention was placed on the way lines relate to each other, forming angles. The words *angle, angel, ankle* and even *ankh* (the Egyptian life force symbol) all share common Sanskrit roots (*anga-m, anka-s*), meaning to curve, bend or hook. This suggests a continuum between body, math and the supernal. The body is linked to the sacred through numbers. The definition of angel, "a messenger bent to earth," bears this out.

Measuring the angles directly formed by the limbs of the *Vitruvian Man* (which, incidentally, Leonardo proportioned in Egyptian cubits), shows **18** degrees, **36** degrees, **54** degrees, **72** degrees, **90** degrees, **108** degrees, and **144** degrees, which are the same angles developed from the five-pointed star form the *Vitruvian Man* mimics—the pentacle. Moreover, the restatement of these angles recurs boldly in Leonardo's early works, such as *Madonna of the Rocks* and *The Last Supper,* and with subtlety in later pieces, such as *Virgin and*

Child with St. Anne, the *Mona Lisa* and *St. John the Baptist* (the muted, slender cross he holds diverges at 72 degrees/108 degrees).

If a mere ratio of the angles proved to be phi, our golden search would end, but simple ratios again won't work, because phi is irrational; 144:90 is 1.6, close but not definitively phi. Yet with the next step, comparing the length or chords (as geometers would identify them) of the pentacle, something instantly lights up. The ratio of a pentacle arm's side to its base is phi precisely. No argument. The arm of the pentacle is thus called a Golden Triangle.

THE FINDER'S PHI

It took a little sleuthing, but the pentacle or rose star (named for its five arms or petals) and its related angles (a.k.a. sacred rose angles) clue us in to the presence of phi. In fact, pentacle angles are an artist's occult reference to phi. A triangle with 72 degrees/36 degrees/72 degrees shows phi when you compare the length of its sides to its base. This same Golden Triangle is pictured as the pyramid on the back of the U.S. dollar bill. America's founding fathers were Masons, an order of golden geometers in existence since the time of King Solomon of Jerusalem.

Pentacle diagrams, though, date back past Renaissance art to Mesopotamian stelae, or columns, revealing their representation in art and architecture for at least 6,000 years, back to the beginnings of hand-baking bread. Critical assessments that artists haven't used phi because their canvases don't measure up in Golden Proportion seem quite beside the point. Using rose angles, an artist can compose an *inner structure* that encodes phi through pentacle association.

Phi is all around us. Pick up a paper, or better yet just the sports section, and find a protractor in the housewares section of the grocery or pharmacy. Put it to the pictures. Check the batting angle of a grand slam or a jump shot, Bode Miller on a carve, a pack of cyclists leaning into a curve: See the rose angles roll. 18 degrees, 36 degrees, 54 degrees, 72 degrees, 90 degrees, 108 degrees, 126 degrees, 144 degrees . . . are the shape of our movement and being. These angles are us! My favorite is a photo of Muhammad Ali tensed (in 108 degrees, 126 degrees and 144 degrees) and dominant after the flooring punch he threw at Sonny Liston in Lewiston, Maine, on May 25, 1965.

Skeletal systems sectioned by phi and a subcellular blueprint based on phi (Israeli biophysicists have discovered that phi programs the width-to-length ratio in each coil of DNA) pretty much make us (and other vertebrates) move in and respond to rose angles.

It seems clear that the art of Leonardo and other Renaissance masters invoked insistent geometry referencing fiveness and the pentacle, using both the indicative messenger angles we've reviewed and through allegorical association with the apple and the rose. Traditional association of phi with the apple and rose is one explanation of why the term Golden Proportion surfaced so recently: In ages past, this sacred harmony was called *ruber* (Latin) or *rudh* (Indo-European)—red!

THE ROSE AND THE CROSS AND THE HEART OF THE MATTER

To this day, we associate red with roses, love, life, emotion and the heart. The heart as an organ has long been considered the crux of life. The rose cross (Rosicrucis) was the mark of a legendary Grail order that protected, discussed, experimented with and implemented crucial information and techniques about the innermost secret workings of life. These rubrics, or "redlined" activities, made their way into the sciences of astronomy, navigation, optics, masonry, physics, medicine and physiology. Rosicrucian members through the ages have included Leonardo, Christopher Columbus and Dante Alighieri; moderns Sir Francis Bacon, Sir Isaac Newton, Ludwig van Beethoven, Benjamin Franklin and Thomas Jefferson; and ancients linking Robert the Bruce of Scots to the Essenes, the Greek Pythagoras, and founder of the order, the Egyptian pharoah Thutmose III. In modern times, we often look at these figureheads as isolated geniuses, but legend has it they were connected through this vital fraternity, which supported and bolstered a particular individual's talents to strengthen the compendium of scientific knowledge amassed through the centuries.

Modern formulae assign phi to the generation of curves; and despite the adage "the shortest distance between two points is a straight line," Einstein's theories and subsequent quantum physics state that any line passing a body of matter *necessarily* bends or warps. A curved, enfolded, implicate universe seems to have been comprehended, quantified and even represented in works of art, architecture, music and literature by the ancients since at least as far back as the construction of the Great Pyramid.

Linguistic delving surprisingly reinforces this theory. *Rose* unexpectedly means dew in Latin and liquid in Sanskrit; the deepest root meaning is to flow. *Cross* is in a family of words with *crisis, crucial, crusade, crucible* and *crux*—all of which we readily identify with central (heartfelt) issues. Again, an unusual tip-off begins with the related word *crosier*, the hooked staff of both shepherd and prelate. The family root definition starts linear, *stake*, but traces back to round pole, further morphs to spine or backbone, then ends in a final twist with the Sanskrit "it curves."

Angle, angel, rose and cross—all associated with the pentacle— *invariably resolve to curves and flow*. This old geometry is far from stiff and is looking and phi-ling (feeling) more like bread dough all the time!

The school of Pythagoras saw such mathematical perfection in the pentacle that they called it *Hygieia,* or health, and used it to represent the five elements: earth, air, water, fire and *hieron*—divine idea or mind. This is the exact formula for bread: grain (earth), leaven (air), water, oven heat (fire) and human intervention through mindful recipes, shaping and timing. The baker knows his hand (pentadactyl) represents this same perennial five-part formula.

There was a further secret meaning—known as *pentemychos*—to the Pythagorean pentacle threading all the way back to Mesopotamia, which translates as angle, nook or hidden chamber. This additional, or sixth, element was the central cavity or heart of the pentacle outlined by the surrounding five Golden Triangle arms. Parallel to the linguistics explored above, this mystical *sex* (the ancient spelling of *six*) space also meant pitfall or place of crisis: a place of cosmic chaos that precedes order and manifestation or the temptation that can undo it. This "gateway to all realms" became known as the Holy Grail, named *krater* by the Greeks from the original Mesopotamian term *graal*. It was the central "curve" of life, represented by a golden crucis (or chalice) together with the red liquid of life it held (represented by blood or wine). The pentacle was therefore both an angular (male) blueprint for phi and symbol for the hidden waters of the sacred female, the primordial sea (Latin *mare*, or mother Mary) out of which flowed all life processes.

From the Renaissance back through the centuries, angles of the pentacle have moved us: The fourteenth-century Moorish Alhambra near Granada, Spain, and Justinian's Hagia Sophia built in 537 CE in Istanbul are indisputable examples of astounding pentacle/phi construction that leave one breathless and weak-kneed. This math of masters—from architecture, alchemy and art to martial movement and dance—turns numbers kinetic and math into movement.

Golden Proportion math is sexy. It's got curves. It turned a cross into the undulation of the backbone. Since I grew up in the 1960s, when Muhammad Ali reigned, I also knew that other king. Get your protractor again, pop in a disc from the man from Memphis and check Elvis's angles. The way he bent his body was banned from sight in many venues of the times. It's not unrelated to why Leonardo's first *Madonna of the Rocks* was rejected in 1493 by the Confraternity of the Immaculate Conception in Milan.

THE STYLUS, *STAUROS* AND THOTH

All modern humans share a single ancestry. We didn't evolve from separate strains, and we never were Neanderthals. Various hominid groups developed the ability to hunt, gather, make tools, build shelter, fashion clothing, make fire and even develop ritualized burial practices—but some animal species exhibit most of these abilities, too.

What distinguished modern man was the capacity to measure, record and remember phenomena—*to keep a recipe*. We made marks that were codifiable, storable and reproducible. Romanian clay tablets impressed with a stylus or hand stake in pre-Sumerian script are our oldest documents, dating to over 8,000 years ago. The earliest writings were logograms, very much like mathematical numerals or musical notation because they were read independently of spoken sounds. They could be pronounced in various dialects or even in entirely different languages and still retain the exact same visual recognition.

Undoubtedly one of the first marks made was the line. A vertical mark might represent man, a tree or pole, or even aspiration. A horizontal line could represent earth, sleep or death. A diagonal line likely related the two (as the words *angle* and *angel* have indeed come to represent).

The upright line on a horizontal base (like an inverted T) could have communicated a signal event: driving a stake into the ground. This was an act of immense scientific import because it created the gnomon, or sundial arm used to calculate time and astrological measure. Eratosthenes of Cyrene correctly determined the circumference of the earth as early as 250 BCE by measuring the angles of shadows cast by large stakes or poles, or *stauros,* sunk into the African earth hundreds of miles apart, 1,800 years before Western Europeans accepted that the earth was round!

The stake, or stauros, became the gnomon or sundial arm that gave rise to circle division, radial geometry and the measurement of time, all credited to a Sumerian god called Thammuz or Thoth. *T* became the sign of Thoth and his teaching, called Tau. From the center of the ancient world (Mesopotamia), the teaching of Tau (Thoth) branched into Tao in the East, which Lao-tsu formalized as the yin/yang principles of the Classic of the Way of Power in China in the sixth century BCE. In the West, his symbol was carried on as the Rose Cross of

Thutmose III ("Born of Thoth") in Egypt in 1450 BCE, then became our cruciform letter *t* and was later assimilated as the modern Christian cross.

Interestingly, the word *stauros* minus the letters of *tau* leaves *s-ros*: not a far stretch from the word Sirius, the ancient Nile Star, which rose helically and marked the Egyptian New Year at summer solstice. This was the time of year when the Nile flooded and deposited its wealth of black mud, which allowed the growing of the famed Egyptian wheat. This most sacred summer month was the month of Thoth.

The year Leonardo died, 1519, marked the last "sighting" of Thoth. Montezuma, the Aztec emperor, mistook Hernán Cortés and the glory of his eleven masted ships for the return of the Great Designer, the lord of the calendar, evolution and sound itself—Thoth, or Quetzalcoatl in Aztec and Mayan lore. Viracocha to the Inca, Teutates in ancient Gaul (France, northern Italy and Germany), and Mercury in the Roman pantheon, Thoth was further recognized even into the thirteenth-century Arthurian Grail stories—renamed as the sorcerer Merlin!

THE HEX OF SUMER

In Leonardo's time, *sex* was a collective term that hadn't yet separated the interaction of the genders. Leonardo's *Mona Lisa* and the sonnets of Shakespeare (a Grail Gnostic himself) reflect this intriguing ambiguity. (Historically, the seventeenth-century poetry of John Donne is considered to be among the first recitals of gender distinction.)

This ambiguity had troubled the church for at least ten centuries, having frighteningly ancient roots that predated the pyramids and dynasties of Egypt to the ancient civilization of Sumer in Mesopotamia, in present-day Iraq.

The sexual or generative power of *six* (the modern spelling of the word) is attached to the most ancient form of that word, *hex*, a word both sacred and cursed. It's a mathematical touchstone—hence its power. Six is the number of sides of the first symmetrical polygon, or angled figure, that can be derived from a circle. This hexagon (restating the sixth element referred to in the pentemychos) was held as the great mother that births the subsequent shapes, numbering 3, 4 and 5—or triangle, square and pentacle.

The Sumerian discovery of this fundamental value of six (or the hex) gave rise to the storied six days of creation (in the Mesopotamian tablet Enuma elish) which was, centuries later, transcribed as the six days of Genesis. Connecting alternate points on the hexagon reveals the six-pointed Star of David, the Masonic symbol of Solomon. The interlocking equilateral triangles produced represent, on one level, the balance and equality of male and female. But deeper, the hex unlocks the 3, 4, 5 sequence of the mystic Masons' triangle made of the rose angles 36, 54 and 90 degrees—in Sumeria 4,000 years before the Greek geometer Pythagoras!

This special configuration keys all Masonic structures, from temples and cathedrals to music and bread. It has also been called the Egyptian triangle or the rope stretcher's right triangle and helped form the duodecimal (base 12) measuring system Americans still cling to $(3 + 4 + 5 = 12)$.

The dizzying potency of this ancient geometry was temporarily unleashed on twelfth-century France in the form of the frenzied building of the Notre Dame cathedrals. Godefroi de Bouillon, traveling under the rose red cross of the Knights Templar, conducted the first and only successful Grail crusade to the Holy Land in 1099 CE. There the buried secrets of Solomon's masons and chemists were unearthed, and this knowledge made the Templars the wealthiest private organization Europe had ever known. They even began the first institution of banking. But after vying for power with the Roman Catholic Church, the organization was believed to have gone underground over a century before the birth of Leonardo.

The real story of the Grail, traceable to the most ancient human municipal society, Sumer, is chiefly concerned with the mysteries of balance and proportion. It reveals a chicken-egg paradox of primacy to the coevolutionary male/female numbers of six and five, also called the lily and the rose (each flower represents that specific number in its petals). This interplay figured heavily into both the structural and emotional power of the work of Renaissance artists.

The everyday stuff of bread symbolizes and embodies this mythic math. The ancient Greeks went so far as to denote the pentemychos as the home of the psyche, or world soul. Making, reflecting on and eating bread restores the commonplace as residence still for the extraordinary.

ALCHEMY AND THE BAKER'S SORCERY

The true alchemical process of making leavened bread seemed to arrive around 3000 BCE from Mesopotamia with the founder of the first Egyptian dynasty, Hor-Aha-Men, or the biblical Ham (or Khem), patriarch of bread. This was the start of the family of bread that included Abra-ham ("come out of Ham"), Solomon and Jesus the Nazarene of Beth-El-Ham ("house of the Lord of bread"), now known as Bethlehem. Their eucharistic (from the Greek word *karizesthai*, to offer graciously) ritual of sharing alchemical bread and wine was famously rendered in a cafeteria mural in 1497 CE when Ludovico Sforza commissioned Leonardo to paint *The Last Supper* for the Dominican monastery of Santa Maria delle Grazie. (The painting was proportioned by what Leonardo termed *secto d'aurea,* or the golden section.)

Ham (or Khem) so influenced Egyptian culture that the country was known because of him as Khemet, translated as "black earth." This also referenced the color of Nile mud, the agricultural wealth left by annual flood, when the Nile rose in the sacred summer month of June—the month of Khem, a.k.a. Thoth. In the Hebrew tongue, Ham (pronounced chaim) equated to Thoth. In the Arabic tongue, whatever came out of the land of Ham was called *al-Khame,* out of Khemet, or "out of the black."

Alchemy (*al-Khame*) referenced all the Egyptian poured arts, from metallurgy and herbal/medicinal infusions to *bedja* bread baking—and shaded them black. The first word for pizza, *picea*, meant "blackened crust." Blackness was reinforced by the Egyptian habit of using the refined ore of antimony, or kohl, to decoratively blacken the eyelids. The Arabic descriptive *al-koh'l* has come down as the sister process to bread baking, the distillation of spirits: alcohol. Barm, or barley beer foam, is often considered the original yeast added to dough to raise bread. Breweries and bakeries existed side by side in Africa five millennia ago.

The processes of shaping materials by fermentation and transformation through fire were cast as black magic or sorcery. Bakers were occasionally taken to be "Merlins"—sorcerers—rising from the mystical association with the pre-deity Thoth. The pyramids are found to be "fire born" also (from the Greek word *pyr* for fire), further sharing a related linguistic root, meaning "inner flame," with the words *heart*, *hearth* and even the word *focus*. The Italian flatbread known as focaccia derives from the Latin *focus panis*. This translates to "hearth bread" or "fire bread."

Making all these ancient secrets known is the work of the modern artisan. Information on its own is near nothing. The application of knowledge through craft sparks fact into flames and fires vitality into human existence.

*E*PILOGUE

SOPHIA'S

The now, the distant cloud. Voices resonating like hands across a fevered brow. Liturgical purple reaching back to Eleusis, where initiates entered the Telesterion to witness revelation. Imagery of grain, or poppy, shown symbolically, possibly carved in marble. Although some theorize real things were preserved & revealed. Treasures rescued by Demeter every spring. Today, I dropped by Sophia's, far enough away from the original Portland Trade Building at 34 Exchange, run by two present-day hierophants, baker/painters, where on Holy Thursday, over all three loaves, for our own small ritual tonight, or as Steve said, "to break," Rick talked of being at Chichen Itza at the exact moment of the equinox ten years ago.

II

Now, I've been at these investigations for a long time. Read practically everything by Karoly Kerenyi, translated into English. When he mentions Eleusis it's a sacred place, *for the survival of personal existence, regardless of death.* How simple, & direct. Steve & Rick's place is that type of architecture the Hungarian scholar alludes to as Sanctuary.

Perhaps he'd even compare it to the Anaktoron, that smaller structure within the larger Telesterion. Maximus of Tyre is quoted to say
that one is not initiated without having reached it. Kerenyi, appropriately enough, compares it to *the chapel of the Porziuncula, in Santa
Maria degli Angeli near Assisi.* Suddenly, ten years ago doesn't seem
that far away.

—ROBERT GIBBONS

For more information on The Diet Code,
Stephen Lanzalotta, and Sophia's, visit
www.diet-code.com.

INDEX